AYURVEDA

The Ancient Indian Art of
Natural Medicine & Life Extension

AYURVEDA

The Ancient Indian Art of
Natural Medicine & Life Extension

BIRGIT HEYN

Healing Arts Press
Rochester, Vermont

Healing Arts Press
One Park Street
Rochester, Vermont 05767

First Quality Paperback Edition 1990

First published in the Federal Republic of Germany in 1983 by Scherz Verlag
under the title *Die sanfte Kraft der indischen Naturheilkunde: Ayurveda*

Library of Congress Cataloging-in-Publication Data
Heyn, Birgit
[Sanfte Kraft der indischen Naturheilkunde. English]
Ayurveda : The ancient Indian art of natural medicine and life extension /
Birgit Heyn.
p.   cm.
Translation of: Die sanfte Kraft der indischen Naturheilkunde.
Includes bibliographical references.
ISBN 0-89281-333-4
1. Medicine, Ayurvedic.   I. Title.
R606.H4913   1990
615.5'3--dc20   90-4040
                                          CIP

Printed and bound in the United States of America

10 9 8 7 6 5 4 3 2 1

Healing Arts Press is a division of Inner Traditions International, Ltd.

Distributed to the book trade in Canada by Book Center, Inc., Montreal, Quebec
Distributed to the health food trade in Canada by Alive Books, Toronto and Vancouver

CONTENTS

PREFACE

The medical system presented in this book is highly likely to promote mistrust of and dissatisfaction with the sort of medicine favored by our industrial society. Naturally, the fundamental differences between the two types of therapy enable us to see with unusual clarity how important are those qualities of life that have been trampled underfoot in the onward march of our civilization.

Ayurveda, one of the oldest systems of medicine known, has managed to preserve its holistic character and to treat man as a complex whole in relation to his environment. Diet and medicinal herbs are among the chief methods it employs for the maintenance or restoration of health. Perhaps it is a thankless task, in such an ecology-minded age, to expatiate once more on the great importance of plants to life on this planet; yet the fact is that we are facing a catastrophe which is not simply something that might happen tomorrow—to some extent it is with us today. Since many negative developments are now seen to be irreversible, since our woodlands are dying because of acid rain, since almost every aspect of life is threatened with a lack of natural qualities, protecting the environment has become a topical political and social issue. Nevertheless, significant improvements are undertaken only when the social consequences become unbearable, just as if the quality of life were nothing more than a question of cost effectiveness.

The need for communication between man and plant, for a restoration of the harmony between people and their environment (which is taken for granted in Ayurveda), has penetrated our consciousness here in the West in a partial and rudimentary fashion. The vegetable kingdom is not indebted to man for its preservation; it is quite the reverse: without plant life man would be unable to exist. Aided by earth, water, and sunlight, plants provide us with our basic raw materials—food and oxygen. They nourish us, keep us healthy, and enable us to overcome our imbalances and diseases.

The chemical multinationals, with their many allegedly vital products, their ultrasoluble fertilizers, their weed killers and insecticides, their growth hormones and hybrid seeds, may produce giant crops but certainly not more or better-quality food. On the contrary, never was there so much hunger or shortage of food in the world as there is today.

What is more, the advertising campaigns of the pharmaceutical industry, according to which beauty comes out of a jar and health out of a bottle, have no connection with reality. Our statistics show a continual rise in the so-called iatrogenic diseases, in which people who only thought they were ill become genuinely ill through overdosing themselves with medications they do not need. They pay dearly for listening to wrong advice, and it is not plants or human health that flourish, but profits. When all is said and done, the ecosystem provides us with abundant materials for nourishing and curing our subtle bodies, but we must re-learn how to perceive nature with all our senses. By outlining the traditional form of Indian medicine known as Ayurveda, the present book should awaken and deepen our understanding of the relationship between man and plant. No claim is being made that this is an intensive course in Ayurveda—such as would occupy at least six years in an Indian university—but medical practitioners of every school and anyone who wishes to live in harmony with nature and to cultivate the full and responsible use of their five senses, anyone who places a high value on body consciousness and inner development, can derive from this book fresh insights and stimulating lines of thought.

It may interest the reader to know how the author came to study Ayurveda. During my pharmaceutical studies, chemistry took pride of place; the main interest of lectures centred on synthetic drugs and their effects. The traditional domestic remedies and the well-tried herbal teas were relegated with a superior smile to the status of old wives' tales. Later on, when working in a pharmacy, I had to sell countless tranquilizers, stimulants, painkillers, pills to take away the appetite, and the like. I could not help being struck by the attitude of the sufferers to their suffering; when selling them some heart or blood-pressure nostrum I realized that scarcely one of them considered his circumstances or way of life or would do more for his health than to swallow a few pills.

This conversion of patients into 'health customers' is part and parcel of the general attitude to medicine in our highly industrialized society, with its rushed consultations in which something is prescribed for each symptom, and with its impersonal hospitals where the human body is treated like a machine waiting for spare parts and a general overhaul, and the human mind is kept on an even keel with psychopharmaca.

Having become disenchanted with what my profession had to offer,

I decided to travel abroad, and during a prolonged stay in Indonesia was introduced by my first teacher, Pak Narso, a master of Tai Chi, to a new way of looking at life. Later on I acquired the basics of Ayurveda at the Hindu University of Benares. The contact with an age-old medical system that made such a splendid showing when compared with our modern schools of medicine incited me to take a greater interest in herbs. I gather and plant herbs, taste, and evaluate them. Admittedly, I had already studied the familiar medicinal plants, but only in the analytical fashion of specialists who try to isolate active principles with cut-and-dried allopathic effects. But now I studied them as a whole, from the point of view of Ayurveda, and in the realization that cures are not effected by exotic wonder herbs but by plants forming part of our immediate environment. The Ayurvedic system is not restricted to certain climatic zones and ecological environments; what interests me now is to integrate the two areas of knowledge: knowledge gained by study and knowledge gained by experience.

I owe a debt of gratitude to my Indian teachers, who in alphabetial order are C.N. Chaturvedi, K.C. Chunekar, P.V. Sharma, S.N. Tripathi and K.N. Udupa.

Without the assistance of Heinz R. Unger in copying the manuscript, this book would not have been possible. He has my warmest thanks.

BIRGIT HEYN

1

THE GREEN POWER OF AYURVEDA
Introduction and Comparisons

All my senses go to work when I am crossing a meadow or tramping through a wood in search of medicinal plants. I feel the fresh air, breathe in the scents of the countryside, note the various shapes and colors, and listen to the humming of the insects and to birdsong gently breaking the deep and blessed silence that is so sweet after the nerve-racking roar of the city. During my hike, I sample various edible berries and often chew a piece of wood sorrel or young dock. I can recognize herbs not only by their favorite habitats, not only by the shapes of their leaves and blossoms, but also by their smell and taste. Our sense of taste is, in fact, very keen. Anything tasted for the first time impresses the memory just as distinctly as something seen or smelled for the first time.

My senses are also busy sending information to my internal warning system. The luscious raspberry is tempting but, sad to say, it grows not far from a motorway. A nearby factory pollutes the atmostphere—the smell is unpleasant and I lose my appetite for wild bilberries and for the dandelion leaves I was going to add to my salad. If a plant is infested by insects, if it is faded and wilted, I no longer want to taste it. These signals from our senses are important for our survival, and we should make every effort to prevent them from being blunted by things put in our food, whether they be chemical preservatives, artificial coloring, or additives to 'improve' the flavor. Yet we are inclined to ignore the senses once the intellect has surveyed our environment and has summed it up in formulas and technical terms.

Plastic flowers do not gladden the heart or dispel troubled thoughts. When diagnoses and indications for therapy are spat out by a computer, the physicians grow rusty, their patients feel unable to make any useful contribution, and the effect of treatment is uncertain.

Earplugs and eyemasks may help the apartment dweller to find sleep in spite of heavy traffic passing his window, but his senses are neither naturally rested nor naturally stimulated—and both things are important.

I see, smell, hear, taste, and feel a person and know whether I like him or her, whether I can love and trust him or her, and whether he or she will be good or bad for me. In just the same way, when I commune with nature, I know which landscape is beneficial to me and which plants I can use. Of course, this requires that I know myself, my temperament, my inclinations, my wishes, and longings; I must also take into account the many external influences and daily conditions. No instrument can provide me with such accurate information on my physical, mental, and spiritual state as is provided by my own subjective consciousness. The apparent objectivity of a perception of the world filtered by technical equipment is essentially inferior to conscious perception.

In Ayurveda we have a medical system which still trusts the human sense organs. *Ayur* means 'life' and *Veda* means 'knowledge'. 'Biology' would be a rough-and-ready translation, but a better rendering is 'the knowledge of how to live.' However, for the benefit of people living in our high-tech civilization, we should expand this to 'the knowledge of how to live naturally.' *Ayurveda* is a knowledge of natural harmony and a method of removing disharmony.

Ayurveda is a form of treatment by natural remedies, which makes use of the powers of nature to restore human beings to a state of balance. The heat of the sun, light, air, and water, and mineral, vegetable, and animal substances (unprocessed if possible) are employed in therapy and as remedies. In addition, Ayurveda has something to say on health education and health preservation. Ayurveda helps us to recognize the correct way to live at a given moment in order to overcome special problems; it helps us, in fact, to anlayze our habits and our environment and to see where we are going wrong.

Well-known and highly prized practices such as meditation and Yoga play an important part in identifying the qualities of a healthy, fulfilled, and aware life. The significance of these spiritual and physical exercises has now been confirmed in the West thanks to the proliferation of a kaleidoscopic variety of psychotherapies and methods of 'bodywork'— the Occidental way of confronting body and mind.

Ayurveda is a holistic medical system, and it has no room for that split between the spiritual and the physical that is part and parcel of our Western Faustian archetype. At the heart of Ayurvedic thinking is the insight that the universe as macrocosm and man as microcosm are in direct relationship, that they reflect one another, and that the one is always present in the other.

This direct link between man and his surroundings is experienced throughout our lives by the use of our senses, which are the instrument of communication. But are we using our senses as originally intended? Are we not handing their functions over more and more to our technical apparatus? How much are we now really hearing, smelling, and tasting the things around us? Is it not true to say that owing to a rapid deterioration in the quality of life we are often discouraged from using our senses to the full, if only to protect them from harmful stimuli? Is it not true that we are increasingly losing contact with the sensuous side of life?

Ayurveda sees an immediate connection between the use of the senses and the origin of disease: *Every wrong use or non-use of the senses leads to a disharmony in man, and to disharmonies between man and nature.* The sameness (*Samanya*) between nature (*Prakrti*) and the self (*Purusha*) is the foundation upon which all the principles of Ayurveda are built.

The balance, the well-being, and the good health of an individual are dependent on the equilibrium of three forces that control all bodily and mental activities. These three forces or principles, the *Tridoshas*, are a reflection of cosmic forces in microcosmic man. The classical Ayurvedic texts describe them in an analogy expressing the original human experience of the forces acting on life. Man is standing on the earth. And there is the sun, there is the moon, there is the wind.

The sun radiates heat and bestows the energy necessary for all physiochemical and biochemical processes. Its representative in man is the force *Pitta*, which controls all the biochemical processes in the body, all reactions resulting in heat, e.g., the digestion of food and cellular metabolism. *Pitta* warms, colors red, and produces the 'glow' of energy in us.

The moon stands in a relationship of tension to the earth; it acts on biological rhythms, rules the tides, and has an affinity with the element water—which is cooling and gives the cells of the body form and firmness. Its representative in man is the force *Kapha*, which has a visible effect in altering the equilibrium of fluids in the tissues and organs and also lubricates the joints. *Kapha* gives the cells, and with them the whole body, form and firmness and has a cooling effect.

The wind not only moves, it *is* the movement of the atmosphere; it blows the clouds along, dries wet places, and sets fires blazing. The motive force in man is the principle *Vata*, the principle of movement. It is the complex nervous system with its impulses. *Vata* is the will to live.

A drought, a forest fire, a flood, or a hurricane bring about a transitory disturbance in the harmony of nature. An increase in *Pitta*, or some disturbance in one of the other principles, will upset the harmony of these three *Doshas* in a living being. Their unstable equilibrium has then to be restored.

The *Tridoshas* are at work in all living creatures. All matter, both animate and inanimate, is taken to be a composite whole made out of five basic elements (the *Panchabhutas*). This essential frame of reference in Indian thought permits a wide variety of relationships between man and his surroundings. It serves to make the relationship between man and plant understandable, since both have been made from the same 'building blocks of existence' and have the same forces working in them, i.e., the same *Tridoshas*.

This relationship was self-evident and important to all the early civilizations; it even seemed to be important for their survival. The shamans of the nomadic races were as familiar with medicinal herbs as were the Egyptian physicians in the 'house of life' on the banks of the Nile. Medicine could be found in the wild, free and without a prescription, and indications for given remedies rested on the experience of many generations. Knowledge consisted of the transmission of this experience. It seems that Ayurveda is the oldest medical system that is still in full use at the present time.

In our highly industrialized and technological society, the pharmaceutical industry has disrupted the ancient relationship between man and plant. We have been left with one or two of grandmother's recipes and with a few tisanes and herbal cures. However there is already a decided swing back to the old ways. People are beginning to take a greater interest in herbs and their uses, and grandmother's remedies are coming into their own again. There is a gradual recognition that it is more in keeping with causal therapy (i.e., with the treatment of causes) to clear up a viral infection such as influenza by perspiring in bed and drinking lime-flower tea than fighting it with antibiotics, or to cure constipation with a change of diet rather than palliating it with laxatives.

Although this is a move in the right direction, we are still being swamped by a huge tide of advertising pouring out from the press and television urging us to believe in the virtues of various tablets, tinctures, ointments, and pills. Our general attitude to pharmaceutical products is no better than that of our benighted ancestors, who parted with good money to fairground mountebanks for various quack cure-alls. We defer to science as if it were a unitary fount of wisdom, whereas it is in reality a number of disciplines often pressed into service by different commercial interests.

In *Das Medikamentenbuch* Paul Lüth writes: 'We take cover in science to such an extent that the section in a firm which sends out leaflets and samples to doctors is known as the 'Scientific Department,' and personnel visiting surgeries and hospitals to explain the advantages of their own firm's products over those of competitors are called 'technical representatives.'[1]

In the logic of our industrialized world, health (like everything else) is a product, and illness is a reduction in productivity. However, our consumption of industrial products as a substitute for our former natural reliance on plants and their virtues is really a sad reflection on the cultural impoverishment brought about by an excessive reliance on technology. The way in which we have relinquished what was once important community knowledge to the hands of a faceless profit-oriented production structure is equivalent to placing this area of knowledge under the control of a trustee—in line with retrograde steps being made in many other social areas.

In India some 70 percent of the population is being treated in accordance with the traditional medical system, Ayurveda, even though 'Western medicine' established a bridgehead there under the British. When we learn that both disciplines are being taught at most Indian universities, we can not help wondering why there has so far been no amalgamation of the two. Ayurveda and the allopathy of industrialized society are poles apart and could be integrated only by a complete change of mind and perhaps by a rediscovery of old truths. Even the simplest concepts such as those of 'health' and 'disease' have different backgrounds and meanings in the two systems.

For example, what do you make of a system of medicine which looks on jealousy, envy, or hate as symptoms of disease requiring treatment? What do you make of a diagnosis in which identifying a specific disease is much less important than recognizing how the patient's total mental and physical condition relates to his environment? And what do you make of a therapy which concentrates on the patient as a whole rather than on his complaint?

In fact, many of these questions are already being aired in the West and are gradually penetrating the consciousness of doctors and patients. The growing disenchantment with technological medicine and with the power of the pharmaceutical industry is accompanied by an encouraging trend towards holistic treatment. A comparative study of an alternative medical system could open our eyes to qualities we have let slip or have never developed. Dr. Hans Harald Brautigam, medical superintendent of a Hamburg hospital and a lecturer at the University of Hamburg, describes a remarkable dilemma: 'Students no longer learn to judge the meaning of such expressions as fear and anxiety on the face of the patient, because they have charts from the path. lab., X-ray plates, computer read-outs . . . No one examines the patient's complexion any more, because reliance is placed on blood counts—not that the latter are unimportant of course.'[2]

Charaka, a classical Ayurvedic writer, defines disease and health thus: 'A disharmony in the constituents which support the body is known as disease, their harmony is called health, the state of normality. A sense of well-being is characteristic of the absence of disease, for disease is always associated with discomfort.'

According to this, Ayurvedic therapy aims not only at healing but also at harmonization; it combats not the illness but the lack of equilibrium. 'Normality' is taken to be the balance of all the constituents of man in harmony with his surroundings. According to a more recent definition, an individual is healthy 'when his metabolism is in equilibrium, he feels mentally well, and his sense organs and motor organs are functioning normally.' On the other hand, an individual is unhealthy 'when he experiences physical or mental discomfort.'

The term *Duka Samyoga*, 'contact with unpleasant things,' means both physical pain and suffering and such emotional disorders as jealousy, anger, fear, avarice, envy, hate, intense feelings, overexcitement, cruelty, and sorrow. 'All these things are afflictions of the mind and body.' Nowadays we have to add the *Duka Samyoga* list such factors as noise and environmental pollution—whether by construction work or by factory waste—and the many forms of poison in our food and other widely used items.

A very similar concept of health is found in homeopathy. As Dr. M. Dorcsi puts it: 'Man is healthy when he is in harmony in himself, with himself, with his environment and with his Creator. In himself because he is holistically intact, with himself because he knows what he wants, with his environment in the social sense, and with his Creator because he has grasped the meaning of life. On this showing, disease is the consequence of an external or internal disturbance of the balance.'[3]

There is a distinct difference in the teachings of official Western medicine and Ayurveda as far as pain and its treatment is concerned. In this connection, Ivan Illich remarks: 'People are forgetting to accept pain as an inevitable part of the conquest of reality, and they interpret each headache as a call to resort to applied science.'[4] In Western practice, pain is killed with medications, narcotics, or medical intervention, the main aim being to fight the disease. In Ayurveda—as in Yoga—'Pain is a help in orientating the unfolding of the Patient's personality,[5] the aim being health education.

The symbol of Ayurveda is the lotus blossom, the eight petals of which represent the eight Ayurvedic disciplines. These disciplines are:

1	*Kayachikitsa,*	internal medicine.
2	*Salya tantra,*	surgery.
3	*Salakya tantra,*	treatment of the ears, nose, throat, eyes, jaws and teeth.
4	*Agada tantra,*	toxicology; the study of poisons.
5	*Bhuta vidya,*	psychiatry; roughly equivalent to the treatment of mental diseases by spirits, mantras, and tantras.
6	*Bala tantra,*	gynecology and pediatrics.*
7	*Rasayana tantra.*	geriatrics; the study of the diseases of old age.
8	*Vajikarana tantra,*	sexology.

As we shall see, surgery developed during the turbulent times of early warfare. In its origins, psychiatry has a certain affinity with shamanistic practices which, as is known, have survived in their pure form in many parts of the world. Child care and female complaints are categorized together to ensure that a sick child is never treated as an isolated individual.

Disciplines seven and eight are concerned with the maintenance of a balanced state in conformity with various requirements, with the object of prolonging life and conserving and increasing potency.

This book can have no pretensions to be a thorough exposition of the entire complex of Ayurvedic medicine, but since a knowledge of curative plants enters into all eight disciplines, a considerable amount of interesting matter has been included. The botanic medicine of Ayurveda, for the most part, employs fresh or dried plants and their natural extracts. This is clearly different from allopathy, which, although it still uses plants, relies mainly on the active principles isolated from them and on standardized preparations. And homeopathy employs highly attenuated, potentized plant tinctures.

Behind every development of a specialized branch of knowledge— whether it be Ayurveda, allopathy, or homeopathy—there is a whole philosophical thought structure with an individual view of humanity and of what goes to make up human life. The core of Ayurveda and of this book is the relationship between man and plant, in other words, 'green power.'

* Translator's note: Other authorities give *Kaumarabhrtya* or pediatrics.

2

I HAVE IT ON THE TIP OF MY TONGUE

Communication Between Man and Plants

Some two thousand seven hundred years ago a certain Jivaka, an ambitious young man whose one desire was to study medicine, made his way to the Punjab, the land of the five rivers, where Prof. Atreya, famous physician and founder of the medical faculty, was lecturing at the University of Taxila. The courses were crowded: for every student who had managed to enroll several more were waiting for a place, and therefore the entrance examinations were stiff. One of the exercises the candidates were set was to go out into the jungle to look for a plant that was medically useless. The young people entered on their task full of hope; its difficulties became apparent to them later. One after the other they returned in a disheartened mood. One, with an air of uncertainty, proferred a weed, another handed over a bunch of prickles, a third brought back a marsh plant, and so on. It was two days before Jivaka reappeared, and then he was empty-handed. He had been unable to find a single plant without some healing power, so he was the applicant accepted. In later years, he became a celebrated specialist in children's diseases and brain surgery.

As this story shows, the classical writers on Ayurveda esteemed the remedial qualities of plants very highly indeed. In our own day and age, we have good reason to cherish their finds. Internationally patented hybrids pose an increasing threat to the old, rich range of varieties, quite apart from the destruction of species being caused by the conditions and effects of our industrial civilization.

Our most effective and strongest remedies still reach us from the vegetable kingdom: for example, the primary glycoside won from foxglove (*Digitalis lanata*), the opiates from the opium poppy (*Papaver somniferum*), colchicine from the autumn crocus (*Colchicum autumnale*), atropine from deadly nightshade (*Atropa beladonna*), aconite from the blue-flowered monkshood (*Aconitum napellus*), reserpine from the Indian snake-bite root rauwolfia (*Rauwolfia serpentina*), strychnine from nux vomica (*Strychnos nux vomica*), and vincristin and vinblastin from the

Madagascar periwinkle (*Vinca rosea*). 'Nowadays we are beginning to rediscover the healing power of plant species which have escaped extinction simply because they survived as ornamental and indoor plants.'[6]

An old Indian proverb puts in a nutshell the difference between the value of plants as food and their value as medicine: 'You do not need medicine if your diet is right, and it is not medicine you need when your diet is wrong.' The meaning is that disease can be overcome by correct eating, and that if eating habits are faulty, even the best remedies can bring no more than temporary relief.

With the population explosion, our planet's food resources are being stretched to the limit. Scientists used to think that food production could be multiplied several times over, thanks to modern developments in genetics and selective plant breading. They talked proudly of a 'green revolution.' Today they are not so sure. After the early triumphs—the initial increase in yields, the breeding of resistant strains, and the adaptation of cultivated plants to various extremes of climate—disillusionment set in as the full extent and severity of the crisis involving food production became apparent.

The breeding of hybrids is still only possible for trained staff at highly specialized institutes belonging to multinationals; these supply the farmer with fertilizers and pesticides, in addition to seed. And that is how the agricultural communities of whole countries have been reduced to a state of economic dependence, for the high cost of seed and chemicals has forced growers in the Third World to concentrate on single crops, for export only, to the detriment of the underfed home markets. Arable land has been ruined by harmful chemicals and erosion, and a rapid increase in the demand for food is aggravated by a global reduction in good farming land and an alarming expansion of desert areas.

The ancestors of nearly all our food plants came from less than a dozen centres where the genetic pool was richly varied. For the most part, these centres lie in the so-called Third World, in regions with harmonious geographical and climatic conditions—the homelands of practically all our most useful plants. Unwarranted interference with these areas is jeopardizing our chances of importing fresh strains from them. In fact, the world's genetic reserves are not being husbanded properly.

When Jimmy Carter, former United States President, commissioned a group of scientists to study trends affecting raw materials and the environment, he received the Report to the President, which became known as 'Global 2000', and the alarming contents of the latter were discussed all over the world. 'Global 2000' had this to say: 'A recently discovered variety of maize provides a dramatic illustration of the catastrophe that could occur if we lose the present rich variety exhibited by the vegetable kingdom. Maize, which is an annual, is cultivated each year at the cost of labor and fossil fuel, not to mention erosion. A plant called Teosinte, related to maize, presumably existed in several varieties, some annuals and others perenniels. If only it were possible to discover a perenniel variety of Teosinte, modern plant-breeding methods might lead to the development of a perenniel maize. Over a period of many years, nothing but annual varieties of Teosinte have been found. Unfortunately, Teosinte grows in only one or two areas in Mexico, where the locals treat it as a weed, and we have to fear that the perenniels—if they ever existed—have been exterminated.'

By a stroke of luck, a student of botany eventually collected a perennial Teosinte plant in a remote Mexican mountain valley. But how many such 'strokes of luck' are we entitled to expect? The report throws a spotlight on the untrustworthy nature of progress when it is misconceived.

In our dealings with nature, our vocabulary has degenerated with our understanding. We no longer communicate with our surroundings, but treat them as not really part of us. Plant specimens (hybrids and others) are turned into articles of commerce, into means of exerting political pressure, into figures in export statistics, into mere objects. We no longer pay due respect to living things and have severed relations with an important part of our life. But perhaps now that we have realized the problem, we shall be better placed to grasp the meaning of 'life with the living', a concept which seemed, and indeed still seems, obvious enough to people of many other cultures. Ayurveda itself starts from the premise that man recognizes and evaluates his environment through his senses: it regards the senses as the door of communication with the environment. For instance, the sense of taste is a bridge for the understanding, a way of estimating the quality of our nourishment in the widest sense.

By making our sense of taste more responsive, by perceiving flavors in a manner special to ourselves, we can learn what things our bodies need. According to science, there are only four flavors the taste buds are capable of distinguishing: sweet, sour, salty, and bitter. Yet this reduced spectrum does not account for everything we actually taste. For one thing, it is necessary to include the two additional tastes taken into the reckoning by Ayurveda, namely pungent and astringent. For another, we are able to detect the consistency of a morsel and can tell whether it is pulpy, crisp, or fatty. We also savor the aroma; and here the nose comes into play, for as is well known, food seems tasteless to anyone suffering from a heavy cold. (Interestingly enough, the old High German word for 'to taste' also meant 'to smell'.)

According to Ayurveda, our daily food ought to contain all six tastes in significant proportions. Sweet foods help body building and energy production; they are found in carbohydrates, fats, and albumen. A certain amount of bitter and sour components in food promotes the secretion of the gastric juices and sharpens the appetite. Many acid substances aid digestion. They contain vitamins, especially vitamin C, and also salts forming the basis of minerals needed to maintain the body's electrolytic balance. Astringents are those foodstuffs containing tannin. They curb overactivity in the small intestine and ensure that the food is digested longer and more thoroughly and is not evacuated too soon.

In due course, we shall learn the exact effects of the different tastes together with their implications for therapy.

3

THE DEEP WELL-SPRING OF THE PAST

Origins and Historical Development

Mankind was driven out of dream time by the blazing scourge of the sun. Climatic changes that set in half-way through the Stone Age and created an inhospitable zone of steadily growing deserts and wildernesses stretching from the Western Sahara to the Kirghiz steppe were the reason for a concentration of populations in the earth's great river valleys. On the banks of the Egyptian Nile, in Mesopotamia, the land of the two rivers, in the Hwang Ho basin in China, and along the Indus of India, advanced cultures developed—the so-called civilizations of the first order. For the first time in history, men were forced to evolve higher forms of social organization. Big cities sprang up as centres of manufacturing, communication, and trade. These crowded places demanded the solution of problems that had never arisen before, including problems to do with the division of labor, stockkeeping, and hygiene.

When the cities of Harappa and Mohenjo Daro were excavated in the Indus valley, an extremely modern-looking system of town planning laid down five thousand years ago was uncovered, with an exact grid of streets, a water supply, sewage, and numerous bathing houses. Obviously, the people of the Indus culture, the dark-skinned Dravidians, appreciated the value of hygiene. Representations of a three-faced divinity* meditating in the lotus position and surrounded by animals were also found. This divinity is thought to be an early form

---

* Translator's note: See also the illustration of a Siberian medal in Vol. V of Maurice's *Indian Antiquities* or Dissertations relative to The Ancient Geographical Divisions, The Pure System of Primeval Theology, The Grand Code of Civil Laws, the Original Form of Government, and The Various and Profound Literature, of Hindostan. This is compared throughout with the religion, laws, government and literature of Persia, Egypt and Greece. The whole work is intended as introductory to and illustrative of The History of Hindostan on a comprehensive scale. Vol. V continues the Investigation of the Oriental Triads of Deity, and details the Horrible Penances of the Indian Devotees. (Published by the author, the Reverend Thomas Maurice, between 1793-1800, London, and sold by W. Richardson under

of the God Shiva, to whom Yoga and the destruction of disease† are ascribed.

The Dravidians were under pressure from wave after wave of nomads streaming down from the region now known as Afghanistan, and were eventually overwhelmed by them. Many of the aboriginal races were driven into Southern India, others were dispersed into the interior of Asia, but some were enslaved by the new rulers. The latter belongs to the Eastern branch of the Indo-Germanic family and were related to the lighter skinned of the Persians. They called themselves Aryan, a word which simply means 'noble'. They spread out from the Indus to occupy the fertile valley of the Ganges and, while doing so, incorporated their pastoral gods and myths of the steppes in the pantheon of the native culture. As overlords, they instituted the oldest and most enduring system of apartheid known to history, which continues to enjoy a *de facto* existence in the Indian caste system. In the beginning there were only four castes. As priests, the *Brahmins* were the spiritual leaders and occupied the apex of the social pyramid. Then came the *Kshatriyas*, the caste of warriors and princes. The caste of *Vaisyas* was that of merchants and administrators. Servants and slaves made up the fourth caste, the *Sudras*, and to this caste the conquered races belonged insofar as they were without rights of any kind.

In the course of time, the main castes broke up, for practical purposes, into many hundreds of subsidiary castes often having a structure similar to that of European guilds of the Middle Ages. Even in present-day India a child can come into the world as a future clothes washer, scavenger, or masseur. The sole difference between past and present is that the old cage of caste is now being exchanged for the new cage of class. Often the bars of the two cages are indistinguishable. What are known as the untouchables still account for the greater part of the population. Mahatma Gandhi wanted to remove the stigma of

the Royal Exchange M.DCC.XCIV.) See also the photograph of the rock carving at Elephanta in Mackenzie's *Indian Myth and Legend* (The Gresham Publishing Company, London, undated but some time between 1912 and 1915. Both Maurice and Mackenzie regarded these three-headed figures are representations of a tri-unity—Brahma, Vishnu, and Shiva according to Mackenzie—rather than of Shiva alone.

† Translator's note: The author says 'medical science', but this veils the sense in which Shiva was supposed to be the god of medicine. As the 'Destroyer' he was 'the destroyer of evil and disease' (Donald A. Mackenzie, *Indian Myth and Legend*, the Gresham Publishing Company, London, undated but some time between 1912 and 1915, p. 148).

untouchability from the pariahs by calling them Harijans or 'children of God.'* To such a 'child of God' it hardly matters what he is called if nothing else changes. In modern India manual work is still despised and is reserved for the lowest castes and the Harijans, who find themselves in the unenviable position of holding all the essential means of subsistence in their hands while being the lowest of the low.

The origin of this development, which goes back to the time of conquest when everything was thrown into the melting pot, is depicted in the classical Indian epic, the *Mahabharata*, beneath the brilliant descriptive power of which there often lie very concrete statements of political realism. Thus the portrayals of the black- or blue-skinned demons, the *Rakshasas*, who were masters of foreign wizardry, hint at confrontations with the dark-skinned Dravidians, whose culture had been driven back into the jungles of the South and who must have known the secrets of the local medicinal herbs, knowledge which in most myths is alleged to confer magical powers.†

What is more, the existence of black gods in the Hindu pantheon— *Krishna* means 'black'—indicates that what we have here is not simply the 'Aryanizing' of an old culture but a cultural fusion in which the conquerors came to terms with the conquered. The water filling the wells from which we draw today comes from many sources.

The stored experience of these races—the distillation of historical, religious, philosophical, and medical knowledge—is found in the four classical Vedas, *Rig Veda*, *Yajur Veda*, *Sama Veda*, and *Atharva Veda*, the origin and date of which remain uncertain, because they were transmitted orally for unknown periods of time before they were ever written down. The four thousand five-hundred-year-old *Rig Veda* and the younger three thousand two-hundred-year-old *Atharva Veda* are important in medical history.

The *Rig Veda*, a collection of one thousand and twenty-eight hymns, gives amazing information on the state of medical knowledge in the ancient world, and mentions operations, the use of prostheses, and sixty-seven medical plants. The *Atharva Veda* documents a considerable further development of the healing art, which, although it rested earlier on a magico-religious basis, offered a whole range of therapies for the most varied diseases, with the help of an impressive armament of herbal remedies.

---

* Translator's note: Literally, 'dedicated to Vishnu.'
† Translators note: But see Mackenzie, *op. cit.*, pp. 70-71, where he argues that '. . . this tendency to identify the creatures of the spirit world with human beings may be carried too far.'

Six of the ablest pupils of the legendary founder of the first school of medicine, *Punarvasu Atreya*, elaborated the medical knowledge of their time in independent treaties. The most notable was written by Agnivesa, and the *Agnivesa tantra* latter formed the basis for the classic work of Charaka. 'The Wanderer' (the meaning of Charaka's name), lived and taught around BC 700 at the medical faculty of the University of Taxila in the Punjab during a culturally peak period. Charaka's book was later revised by Dridhabala but retained the title *Charaka Samhita*, takings its place as the first fundamental medical text.

The second pillar of classical Ayurveda, the *Susruta Samhita*, was erected about a hundred years after Charaka by Susruta, who was one of Divodasa's scholars. Divodasa, a king of Kasi, the present-day Benares, obviously knew how to combine politics and science, since he improved his surgical knowledge mainly by the study of war injuries. Susruta made a compilation of the whole of medical knowledge, with special reference to surgery. This was the *Susruta Samhita*, which is still consulted today.

The advanced civilizations of the ancient world quite clearly cross-fertilized one another. They were linked by trade routes, and there was a leisurely exchange of ideas, which, within several generations, produced far-reaching progress. Thus we have the *Codex Hammurabi* for Mesopotamia and the *Papyrus Ebers* from Egypt some two hundred years younger (each bearing comparable witness to the state of medical knowledge), both antedating the *Atharva Veda*, although they are not as old as the *Rig Veda*. So different cultures were developing along parallel lines in the Vedic era, and it is possible if not probable that they made fruitful contributions to one another. It is also possible, indeed highly likely, that Hippocrates, who lived some two hundred years after Susruta and three hundred years after Charaka, possessed at least a rudimentary knowledge of the fundamental medical works of other parts of the world. Charaka and Hippocrates were the 'fathers of medicine' in their respective civilizations. Now, when we recall that during the cultural flowering of the Han dynasty about BC 200 medical knowledge went through a remarkable period of expansion in China, too, we cannot help being impressed by how short a time it took, historically speaking, to lay the foundations for a further development of the healing art in all the main centers of human endeavour.

When Darius, around BC 500, spread the Persian sphere of influence into the Indus valley, the artifices of war and subjugation were just as unpleasant as at any other period, but the upshot was a fruitful and effective exchange of knowledge and experience between the different cultures. Then again, the incursions of Alexander the Great some two hundred years later were as barbarous as any other raiding parties in the history of mankind, but in many ways they had the character of a scientific expedition such as had never been undertaken before. The fund of knowledge possessed by the great civilizations multiplied rapidly within a relatively short space of time. Not only did the sciences grow away from their magico-mythical roots in order to become more empirical, but philosophy, art, and religion also thrived.

When Buddha, a member of the Kshatriya caste who was born about BC 550, started teaching that each man can find his own way to salvation, he made a direct attack on the leading position of the priestly Brahmins; in other words, he was waging a 'caste war.' Three hundred years later or thereabouts, King Asoka—a Kshatriya warrior who had carved out for himself a stable kingdom from the Hindu Kush to the Bay of Bengal, from Kashmir to Mysore—renounced Hinduism and made Buddism the state religion. Under Asoka, hospitals were founded up and down the land, doctors and nurses were trained, herb gardens were planted, and medical knowledge became a most formidable weapon in the hands of Buddhist monks as they proselytized throughout Asia. The medical system spread with Buddhism, and Ayurveda or one of its offshoots is still being practiced today in Tibet, in Central Asia, in Sri Lanka, in parts of China and Japan, and in Indochina and Indonesia.

Because Ayurveda was so widely disseminated, the Sanskrit texts were translated into many different languages. Consequently, treatises were preserved in the cooler climatic regions, such as Tibet and Nepal, long after the Sanskrit originals had perished, with the happy result that the originals could be reconstructed. In 1890, Lieutenant Bower, a British army officer, discovered in the ruins of Mingat in Eastern Turkestan a mysterious manuscript consisting of fifty-one birch-bark leaves. This 'Bower Manuscript' is one of the oldest medical texts to survive, the legacy of an itinerant monk of the time of Asoka, a specialist in Ayurveda who had noted down the qualities of the tastes and their effects on the *Tridoshas*, the three forces governing all biological processes.*

The fact that the Ayurveda system was able to prove its worth in the most varied climatic conditions was another reason for its spreading so successfully.

---

* Translator's note: The three *Doshas* are, strictly speaking, 'three faults,' or unbalanced conditions of the three *Dhatus*, and it is the latter which are the 'supporters' of the body.

The first centuries of our present era seem both in the Asiatic and in the Mediterranean cultures to have been periods during which the works of the ancient masters were elaborated and extended, quite irrespective of contemporary political movements. In the Roman Empire, the celebrated Doctor Galen made a systematic study of traditional medical knowledge, and in India, the third pillar of the classical Ayurvedic triad was erected, a two-volume work comprising the *Astanga Samgraha* and the *Astanga Hridaya*, which synthesized the works of Charaka and Susruta and formed a digest of the eight parts of Ayurveda in prose and verse. The authors of this impressive and comprehensive production were Vagbhata the elder and Vagbhata the younger.

The Middle Ages, too, show a parallel development taking place in very disparate cultures. While the alchemists of Europe were seeking the elixir of life and the formula for a chemical process that would enable them to manufacture gold and hitherto unknown substances artificially, Nagarjuna and his school in India were investigating the medicinal properties of minerals and metals and were developing methods of preparing mineral and metallic remedies. A formula for which many a Western alchemist might have sold his soul to the devil, i.e., directions for manufacturing gold, can actually be found in the medieval Ayurvedic texts; however, little is made of it, since the process is so complicated and costly that ordinary gold is far less expensive.

When the Moguls set up their empire and brought it to its high point in the fifteenth and sixteenth centuries, the might of Islam overlaid the rich mosaic of religions in the subcontinent. For the traditional medical science of Ayurveda, this meant a period of stagnation and repression as the Moslems introduced their own system of healing, *Unani* medicine. The name is a corruption of 'Ionic' medicine, Greek medicine being one of the main bases of the highly evolved Islamic medical system. Even the Europeans of this era acknowledged that the best physicians were practicing in Arab lands. One of the most celebrated of the hakims, Avicenna [Abu 'Ali ibn Sina], wrote *al-Qanun* (The Canon of Medicine), a compendium of the opinions of Hippocrates and Galen in a new form; this was to remain the most important medical work for the next five hundred years.

Looking now at the changing relationships between the Mediterranean world and the Indian cultures, it is interesting to see how these relationships turned full circle. Unani medical science was an importation not of alien knowledge but of cognate knowledge. In the India of today, Ayurveda, Unani, and Western medicine are practiced side by side, and in the India of the day before yesterday ruled by the

Moguls, there was a fruitful exchange of ideas and a mutual enrichment of the two old healing systems in spite of Islamic dominance.

At the beginning of modern times, the last great work of the so-called Ayurveda classics was written, the *Bhava Prakasa*. Its author, Bhavamisra, an important physician from Benares, introduced many fresh aspects into the time-honored system and supplied information about numerous herbs not known to the ancients. Mercury was first used as a remedy at this time, and indeed on a poignant occasion. In 1498 the Portuguese landed on the Malabar coast and set up trading stations, built forts, and eventually founded colonies, bringing with them syphilis, among other dubious gifts from the lands beyond the setting sun.

If the Portuguese were mainly interested in secure trading posts, the British, who followed them with the establishment of their East India Company in 1600, laid claim to sovereignty of a very different order. They won support from the indigenous oligarchy, played on the rivalries of the various racial groups, and added practically the whole of the subcontinent to their world-wide collection. The expressions of native culture were suppressed or were put under glass in the British Museum. In 1833 the East India Company, having seen fit to give India the benefit of Western science, closed and banned all Ayurveda schools and opened in Calcutta the first university for Occidental medicine. This cultural arrogance on the part of the colonists was apparently encouraged by the revolutionary changes that had taken place in Western medicine in the eighteenth century. The narrow limitations imposed by the standard of knowledge of the Middle Ages had been transcended; hoary old theories had been laid to rest, and a chain reaction had been set off which was similar to those occurring in natural philosophy, technology, and industrialization.

In the machine age, medicine was regarded from a new and special point of view. When William Harvey discovered the circulation of the blood (which had already been described by the Ayurveda classical writer Susruta), the spirit of the age led men to assume that our bodies are machines in motion. Jacques Attali has pointed out the distorted thinking in our present-day medical theories that is ascribable to this way of looking at things: 'In the metaphor of the body as a machine, disease is a breakdown, or an interference with proper functioning; it is seen as a neutral, objective entity, capable of being analyzed without reference to the patient's position in society, and is therefore always open to the same treatment whatever the state of the body concerned. Thus defined, illness becomes a thing apart from the body that is ill.'[7]

Whereas all medical systems used to resemble one another, there came a parting of the ways that was both new and dangerous in the history of mankind. From that portentous moment, the medicine of industrial civilization has been eminently different from all other medical systems. The medical schools of industrialized countries were caught in the general trend and became handmaids of the 'sciences.'

Only in recent years have several mental shutters been timidly opened in order to re-admit some rays of light. Psychosomatic disorders, for instance, are being taken more seriously: the connection between physical and mental factors in the course of disease is acknowledged, and here and there—though as yet they are few and far between—we have hospitals with psychosomatic departments. Homeopathy and anthroposophic medicine are tolerated and are found worthy of discussion. Foreign therapies such as Chinese acupuncture and various types of massage have also been integrated with Western medicine, but often without any real comprehension of their spiritual background.

The fresh approach to the problem areas of pregnancy and parturition, with its slogan 'easy childbirth,' is further evidence of a change for the better. An increase in the number of home deliveries is restoring the view that childbirth is not a disease but a natural process.

There is also a growing awareness of unknown regions stretching well beyond the territory ruled by technology, regions which cannot be mapped out according to current systems, yet are important because of their practical use.

4

THE SHAPING OF THE FUTURE
Things Present and To Come

In colonial days, Ayurveda sank in India to the status of 'poor man's medicine.' Only those who had no money for Western treatments slipped quietly into the hut of an Ayurveda doctor, who might have been a complete charlatan. The knowledge survived, but it had no prestige. Industrial civilization held a fascination, and Western medicine's slapdash way of treating isolated symptoms appealed to people.

As Indians began agitating for independence, they also looked back to their own cultural heritage, and Ayurveda experienced a revival. When I was studying at the Hindu University of Benares, I took an interest in the history of this institution, bound up as it is with the progress made by the Ayurveda system during the present century. The university was founded in 1916 by Shri Malvia with the help of Annie Besant, the theosophist, and its aim was the preservation of the cultural heritage. At first, Ayurveda was taught in the faculty of Oriental Studies and Theology, and each Ayurveda student was also a Sanskrit scholar. Then in 1928 Ayurveda was given its own faculty. In 1963 the Faculty of Indian Medicine became part of 'modern medicine' because of the persistent desire to combine the two medical disciplines. Today the Ayurveda students also learn Western diagnosis and therapy; yet in spite of some positive exchanges of ideas, the contradictions between the two systems are unresolved.

I have observed that there are nowadays two schools of thought among Ayurveda doctors. While one kind of doctor relies entirely on the classical precepts of Ayurveda, the other kind will accept nothing that cannot be proved by modern science. This demand for proof, understandable and desirable though it may be, does become a problem if it is made the sole criterion; for the implied doubt as to the value of direct perception through the senses and the refusal to use intuition, our 'sixth' sense, is abandonment of a vital feature of Ayurveda. Science and technology should be our tools, not replacements for personal knowing and feeling.

At the present moment, Ayurveda is enjoying yet another revival. In the course of the last ten years, medical men in increasing numbers have come to India from all over the world to investigate various aspects of Ayurveda. This growing interest has naturally reinforced the prestige and self-esteem of the Indian experts. In 1983 the first International Ayurveda Congress was held. In September 1978 a conference of the World Health Organization of the United National (WHO) held in Alma Ata, U.S.S.R., addressed itself to the problem of medical care in the so-called developing countries, and concluded that Ayurveda would be the most helpful system for these countries, since it can be practiced in a self-sufficient manner in any climate, and since it reduces the dependence of the poorer nation on industrial states and on the multinationals (especially those involved in the pharmaceutical industry).

The latter aspect will seem even more significant when we realize that the thirty largest multinational drug companies are currently shipping about a third of their exports to the Third World. In a study made of the business practices of the pharmaceutical multinationals, the Swiss political economist Marcel Bühler pointed out that certain medications, which in the lands where they are manufactured have had to be taken off the market owing to their dangerous side effects, are still being distributed in the developing countries.[8] Whereas in the industrial countries legal restrictions and stringent labeling requirements ensure at least some degree of control over the pharmaceutical market, commercial interests in other parts of the globe are often in the hands of corrupt regimes. And so it happens that one of our well-known drugs can dramatically change its stated sphere of application when it arrives in a developing country.[9] Anabolics, for example, which stimulate muscle growth but are a serious long-term health hazard, are recommended for 'underweight' and 'serious protein deficiency.' Western pharmaceuticals often turn out to be harmful in the tropics. For example, remedies for diarrhea (a common ailment in those parts) may appear to work well but aggravate the underlying condition.

In 1978 the WHO drew up a list of the absolutely essential medications, 240 in all. This 'Essential Drug List' of the World Health Organization angered the pharmaceutical industry, and the professional association of the drug companies, the IFPMA, protested vigorously against the 'interference with competitive marketing.'[10] Their competing lines total thousands upon thousands of special preparations. Even at the Ayurveda Hospital in Benares, pharmaceutical representatives queue up daily waiting to hand out their samples.

But the upper and middle echelons of society in the poorer lands of the world are not just one big market; they also have a valuable raw material called 'knowledge' to offer—old knowledge and young workers. Prestigious drug companies have transferred their research departments to India. The French magazine *Le Nouvel Observateur* quotes a Swiss pharmacologist as saying: 'This land (India) is overflowing with highly qualified scientists. They have to accept salaries well below Western standards.'

However, this lucrative aspect cannot entirely explain the increased interest of the multinationals in lands of the Third World. There is another component—the treasures awaiting discovery. Numerous Western pharmaceutical companies have studied the immensely rich plant life of India in an effort to isolate unknown active principles.

When the Indian botanist Virbala Shah, acting on behalf of the great West German multinational company, Hoechst, which had been funding a research center in the neighborhood of Bombay since 1972, went scouring the remotest corners of the subcontinent in search of medicinal herbs, she took her cue from indications contained in Ayurvedic literature.[11]. After isolating the active principles of such herbs, the researchers endeavor, by altering the chemical structure or by total synthesis, to develop substances which will combat tropical diseases or diseases of the heart and circulation. The enormous outlay involved has been justified by the many successes. Thus from the turnip-shaped root of *Coleus foscolii* 'Foskolin' has been isolated; it is able to intensify heart muscle contraction and acts as a hypotensive. From *Stephania glabra*, which Virbala Shah had brought back to the laboratory some ten years previously, a modified active principle was eventually developed which dilates the peripheral blood vessels, is hypotensive, and acts as a prophylactic against infarction.

Some two hundred medicinal Indian plants a year are being tested in the research laboratories of the multinationals, or about eighteen hundred plants to date. If it is possible to isolate from the plant extract an active principle, the latter is chemically analyzed to discover how the atoms of its component molecules fit together and then, after clinical trials, synthetic copies are put on the market as a new money-making product. Although a new product of this kind has its roots in Ayurvedic knowledge, its synthetic form is dictated by the theories of industrialized medicine and has nothing to do with genuine Ayurveda.

Meanwhile, many of the developing countries have been taking steps to lessen their dependence on the multinational drug companies. Some have started creating their own pharmaceutical industries; others, such as Peru and Sri Lanka, have banned the use of trade names and have set up state vending organizations to buy generic drugs from the cheapest suppliers in the world market. These drugs are labeled simply by their chemical code names.

As an active member of the WHO, Bangladesh, one of the poorest countries in the world, has adopted a recommendation made by the World Health Organization and has issued a new drug control order forbidding the importation and use of more than 1700 medications considered by its Ministry of Health to be useless, harmful, or too expensive.[12] Eight multinational companies in Britain, France, Germany, Holland, and the United States are affected by the ban and have responded with a campaign against the health policy in Bangladesh, even though 70 percent of the drugs concerned have been classified as worthless or dangerous by American and European authorities, too. A catalog of 150 preparations has been drawn up for Bangladesh as sufficient for treating disease anywhere in the country. These preparations are now being manufactured for the state and are 50 percent cheaper than their brand-name equivalents.

Since there is a growing tendency for developing countries to rid themselves of their dependence on a world market serving the interests of the highly industrialized countries, Ayurveda is bound to become more important in the future. Therefore, in summing up, I should like to underline once more its distinctive qualities:

- Ayurveda is a 'life science' in the truest sense and lays great emphasis on preventive medicine, including proper nourishment, hygiene, and a safe drinking-water supply. No pharmaceutical company is needed for any of these things.
- Ayurveda does not give the patient local treatments of individual organs, but treats him as a whole. The pharmaceutical companies, on the other hand, mainly supply specifics.
- Ayurveda uses animal, vegetable, and mineral substances taken from the immediate natural environment, and the preparation of the remedies is simple and inexpensive. Imports are unnecessary, and there is no need for foreign advisers or loans.
- Ayurveda remedies act on the total body, strengthen the powers of resistance, promote healing, and have no poisonous side effects.

5

CREATION AS AN ON-GOING EVENT
The Spiritual Background

'Each individual is the unique expression of a recognizable finely tuned cosmic process occurring in time and space.' This is how the writer of the *Charaka samhita* understands the fundamental relationship between a man or woman and the world. Human life is seen as a note in the cosmic harmony. The individual, who is a 'one-off', a once-only, unrepeatable event, exists as a microcosm in the macrocosm of Being. The two systems, human and cosmic, are linked permanently, since both are built from the same basic elements. All the elements contained in the macrocosm are also present in the microcosm.

It is on this spiritual basis that the edifice of Ayurveda has been raised, and theory has been turned into practice. A knowledge of the basic elements, the building blocks of all that is, makes it possible for us to classify materials (including medications by their properties). These perceptible and classifiable properties are perceived through the five senses, which, according to the teaching of Ayurveda, enable us to make subjective contact with the objective universe. The five human senses correspond to the five fundamental elements out of which everything that exists is constructed. These building blocks, called *Mahabhutas*, are present in every substance in different proportions and forms of expression. Dominant elements are easily recognized by their characteristic properties and, with care, the different material combinations can be distinguished.

Each of the great human cultures has put forward its own version of the idea that all things consists of some such fundamental elements and, although they may not have agreed on the number or kind of these elements, they have certainly agreed on the correspondence between microcosm and macrocosm and on the factual coherence of all that is. What is special about the Indian way of looking at things, however, is that it makes no bones about assuming a direct, physical relationship between man and the universe: There are five senses and five perceptible 'building blocks of being'. Thanks to its inherent soundness, this hypothesis of two interlocking systems has held its own for thousands of years in the face of every doubt and philosophical investigation.

The Indians did not develop theology as we think of it in order to explain existence and how life began; instead they interwove strands of mythology and philosophy, both spun on the same spindle. Of the six orthodox philosophical systems derived from the *Upanishads*,[13], only the two oldest have any significance for our study. These are the *Nyaya-Vaisesika* and *Samkhya*. In essence, Ayurveda is no more than the application of these philosophies to everyday life. *Nyaya-Vaisesika* is a doctrine of categories rather than a philosophy, and insists on the reality of the different objects of knowledge listed by it. *Samkhya* philosophy derives from the most ancient sources and explains the structure of the world in terms of a theory of transformation. This very early attempt to account for the universe, which does not acknowledge a creator or any act of creation (apart from the implied principle of continuous creation)*, explains the existence of matter as a mutual relationship between two basic principles: *Purusha* and *Prakrti*.

Prakrti is matter in the widest sense of the word: it is unmanifest, unconscious nature, the womb of physical and biological development in the universe and an all-embracing dynamic principle. *Purusha* is taken to be consciousness in its widest sense, the universal spirit principle, eternal and incorporeal.[14]

Out of the field of tension between the conscious but undynamic spirit principle and the unconscious but dynamic matter principle 'the all' is continually arising. The two principles cannot be transmuted into one another; they simply act on one another and so operate jointly. In this continuous act of creation, the spirit principle remains unaltered; only the matter principle undergoes transformation, because this principle is in unstable equilibrium when in an energy-packed state of tension.

The matter principle possesses three qualities, three leading properties known as *Gunas*, whereas the spirit principle is without such qualities. The matter principle preserves a balanced tension between its three leading qualities. This is its original condition: a pre-creative stage. But the spirit principle intervenes to disturb that balanced tension and causes matter itself to appear, the form in which it appears being determined

---

* Translator's note: The theory of 'continuous creation' still has its adherents, but most scientists have accepted the 'big bang' theory, according to which the universe instantly exploded into being and became diversified as it expanded and cooled.

by the relative strengths of the three leading qualities.

Now the *Gunas*, or three leading qualities of the matter principle, are the cosmic elements known as *Sattwa*, *Rajas*, and *Tamas*. *Sattwa*, or 'essence', represents refinement, the fine structure of substances, and is a reflection of 'otherness', of the spirit principle in the material world, the well-spring of consciousness. *Rajas* is the quality of dynamics, of alteration and change. It is the basis of energy itself. *Tamas* represents the 'dark' quality of inertia and resistance; it represents what is coarse, rough, and heavy in matter.*

These three imperishable basic qualities of the matter principle cannot be separated from one another nor are they operative on their own. Only through the presence of the spirit principle can there be any manifestations of matter as one of the three qualities becomes more prominent and the two others become correspondingly weaker.

It is in this way that *Samkhya* philosophy explains the coming into being of the physical world. There is no disguising the fact that any attempt to interpret this venerably old yet perennially young system of thought is bound to end up as an unsatisfactory paraphrase. The associations evoked by words form part of a whole cultural heritage. To be able to enjoy fruit plucked from the Indian tree of knowledge we need to appreciate the meaning of the tree. Possession of a wide range of the relevant associations is required before we can fully understand each term; we can understand, for instance, that if the three properties of the matter principle are applied to the thought life, *Rajas* becomes the quality of doubt, *Tamas* becomes error or delusion, and *Sattwa* becomes probability.

But where does life fit into this admittedly abstract scheme of primary creative forces? And where do we humans fit in? With the spirit principle acting as a catalyst, any disturbance of the unstable equilibrium of the three basic properties of the matter principle sparks off a chain reaction bringing about the manifestations of *Buddhi*, *Ahamkara*, and *Manas*, three psychic qualities also referred to in the ancient texts as the 'three inner organs'. These stand in an unbreakable relationship with one another and together build the human psyche. *Buddhi* is the intellect, *Ahamkara* the ego, and *Manas* the mind or spirit. *Buddhi*, one might

---

*   Translator's note: Bhagavan Das, in *The Science of the Self*, (Bhagavan Das, The Indian Book Shop, Benares, 1938) suggests that these terms 'may be rendered in English, more appropriately perhaps than by any other triplet of words', by cognisability, movability, and desirability, adding that in a concrete piece of matter they become quality, movement, and substance, which are, respectively, the objects of cognition, action, and desire.

say, represents the switching center of our 'internal computer,' controlling both ego and psyche and also the sense organs, the experiences of which are converted into knowledge by the intellect. This 'inner organ' stores, works out, infers, remembers, and is at the same time the receiving station of the unconscious. It imparts a direct awareness of self. The ego, *Ahamkara*, is the organ that shapes the personality. The three qualities of the matter principle, when in a state of imbalance, have a fundamental formative influence on the personality and imprint themselves more or less strongly on the character according to their several strengths at the time.[15] *Manas*, for which we have no better word than mind or spirit, is the sense organ of inner perception.[16]

In addition to the internal organ *Manas*, there are also five sense organs and five executive organs under the control of the 'spiritual' *Guna*, *Sattwa*, and influenced by the 'dynamic' *Guna*, *Rajas*. Corresponding to these subjective manifestations are others that are objective, being manifestations in the world (the ego's opposite number). By this we mean that under the control of the 'material' *Guna*, *Tamas* and influenced by the dynamic *Guna*, *Rajas* are the five finer and five coarser elements of perception; the latter combine in many complex ways since they are building blocks of every piece of matter.

The five human senses—smell, taste, sight, touch, and hearing— answer to the five elements of perception: scent, flavor, form and color, consistency (palpability), and sound. The five executive organs are the hands, feet, genitals, anus, and tongue. The five primal elements, the fundamental building blocks of being are earth, water, fire, air, and ether (*Prthivi, Jala, Tejas, Vayu, Akasha*).

The three fundamental qualities of the matter principle produce the distinctive properties of the primal elements. *Tamas* gives rise to the element earth; *Tamas* and the psychic quality *Sattwa* give rise to the element water; then again, *Sattwa* and the dynamically acting fundamental quality known as *Rajas* give rise to fire; the element air is brought into being by *Rajas* and, finally, the element ether is brought into being by *Sattwa*. In fact, all three of the fundamental qualities or *Gunas* are present in all of the elements, but the disturbance of the equilibrium has given a fixed dominance to one or two *Gunas* in each element. The Hindus explain the trinity of the *Gunas* in the following way: 'Brahma creates the universe through *Rajas*, Vishnu preserves it through *Sattwa*, and Shiva destroys it through *Tamas*.[17]

Strictly speaking, the 'principle of light,' *Sattwa*, signifies goodness; the 'gloom princple,' *Tamas*, signifies darkness; and *Rajas* signifies dust, perhaps as a symbol for the life energy fluctuating between light and darkness in clouds of passion and uncertainty.

The harmony of the macrocosm has its counterpart in the microcosm, in man. From this point of view, Ayurveda is a theory of harmony.

The following chart simplifies these principles of the spiritual backgrounds.

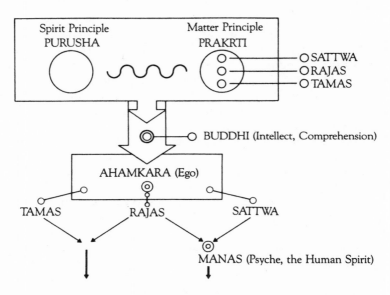

Elements of Perception
Scent
Flavor
Form, color
Consistency
Sound

Basic Elements
Earth
Water
Fire
Air
Ether

OBJECTIVE SIDE

Senses
Smell
Taste
Sight
Touch
Hearing

Executive Organs
Hands
Feet
Genitals
Anus
Tongue

SUBJECTIVE SIDE

6

THE BUILDING BLOCKS OF EXISTENCE
Immediate Perception Through the Senses

'The five building blocks of existence are the point of conflict between philosophy and Ayurveda—the practical application of knowledge. In tracing the origins of the primary elements philosphy is supreme, but in their development the supremacy belongs to science.'[18]

Earth, water, fire, air, and ether—in the spectrum of all their shades of meaning they are quite simply the universe. Everything that has being—a landscape, a plant, a man or woman, or whatever—everything is made from these building blocks of existence.

Each of our five senses is understood to be the main organ of perception for a specific basic element. Of course, no element ever appears in its pure form; the others are always intermixed with it. Nevertheless, one always predominates and leaves its imprint on matter. Similarly, all the senses are involved in each act of perception, but one of the senses takes the lead in perceiving the effects of a particular element.

Thus the element air is perceived by the sense of touch. We may see how branches bend in the wind, we may sniff the scent of the breeze, but most of all we feel the pressure of the air flow on our skins. Yet it is also true that we can perceive any other of the elemental forms by means of our sense of touch. The Ayurvedic classical writer, Charaka, offers this description of the building blocks of existence: 'The main characteristic of Earth is roughness, that of Water is fluidity, of Fire heat, of Air expansion and of Ether a complete absence of resistance. All these characteristics can be detected by the sense of touch.'* So then, we can burn our fingers in the fire, but the main perception of fire is the seeing of its light.

The sense of smell is our principle means for perceiving the element

---

* Translator's note: We should avoid accepting such lists of descriptions as definitive. Much depends on the point of view. Another list, for example, assigns expansion to fire and not to air, and informs us that air is characterized by locomotion.

earth. This association may strike Westerners as rather farfetched, because we have almost forgotten the smell of the soil. But when the monsoon rains fall on the broad, fruitful plains of India after the dry season, the origins of the association becomes clear. The well-soaked earth is perceived by all our senses, but most arrestingly by the sense of smell.

The 'building block', water, is perceived by the sense of taste. Taste is very important in Ayurveda, because it is the means used to make an accurate estimation of the properties of medicinal plants and other substances. Its connection with the liquid element is evident even in the organic sphere, since a flow of saliva is generally necessary before anything can be tasted.

Hearing is the main sense associated with the element ether. Radio waves carrying spoken messages 'through the ether' provide a helpful analogy here.

All our senses play a part in our perception of the world, but what we perceive through them is not the abstract existence of a building block of being but its typical and unalterable fundamental properties.[19] These are what make our perceptions differ from one another. The fundamental properties of the elements show us what the world really is.

An array of ten contrasted pairs of basic qualities is adequate for enabling us to define our precepts. Examples of such contrasted pairs are cold-hot, hard-soft, and rough-smooth. Ancient sources mention a larger number of contrasting pairs, but the usual set of twenty is perfectly adequate. A special advantage of this set of simple descriptive words is that it can be understood without any distortion of meaning wherever it goes; even in translation the words evoke practically the same associations the world over.

The qualities assigned to the building blocks of existence are tried-and-tested descriptions of how a given element will reveal itself. Earth can be heavy, hard, dry, static, slow, solid, or coarse. Water can be liquid, sticky, mobile, cold, soft, heavy, or slow. Fire can be hot, dry, quick, fine, light, coarse, and clear. Air can be fine, light, and clear but also dry and cold. And ether is smooth, fine, soft and clear.*

Any impression of a given substance is the sum of its specific qualities. The manifold nature of existence reaches us through our five senses, and the preceding basic list of what our senses perceive enables classical

---

* Translator's note: This listing differs slightly from the more accurate one later in the book, where fire is smooth (not coarse), air is mobile (not cold), and ether is light (not smooth).

Ayurveda to make accurate assessments in virtually every area. So, for example, there are five typical types of landscape, corresponding in structure and vegetation to the basic building blocks of existence.

A predominantly 'earthy' landscape (*parthiva*) is stony, hard, and blackish, an almost treeless waste. A 'watery' landscape (*apya*) is cool and gently sloping, is found near a body of water, and has carpets of tender herbs and fields waving with grass and corn. The old texts swarm with descriptions of landscapes of this type. The 'fiery' landscape (*agneya*), on the other hand, is rocky; its soil and rock display many different colors, and there are just a few, pale-colored trees and grasses. An 'airy' landscape (*vayavya*) is rough and dry, ash-colored or grey, and supports only a few exceptionally hardy plants. The 'ethereal' landscape (*akasiya*) is soft and erratic, with pure, clear water and high mountains mantled in luxuriant vegetation. The trees belonging to this landscape contain small-sized heartwoods.

When confronted with this simple yet effective system of definitions, we Westerners are liable to look down at it because we so are used to other patterns of thought. Accurate descriptions of the environment are part of everyday life in an industrialized society. Practically everything is measured, weighed, and analyzed. Everywhere we look we are surrounded by instruments unceasingly supplying us with exact data: clocks, speedometers, thermometers, hygrometers, etc. Radio and TV bombard us with time checks, tide tables, weather forecasts, and countless other facts and figures. The precise composition of each bar of chocolate is marked on the wrapper, and the active constituents of each bottle of medicine are printed on the label. Our way of looking at the world through a mesh of crisscrossing data has given us the comforting idea that modern man is in firm control of his environment, thanks to science and technology.

In fact, progressive developments are showing with increasing clarity that the reverse is true, and things are not turning out as originally intended. We are steadily losing contact with the real world. Can we still read the face of nature? Are we still properly aware of our bodies? We are neglecting the use of our five senses and in doing so are letting go of our most natural set of instruments for examining the world. What we are now for the most part experiencing is not the world itself but a technically filtered picture of the world.

The technical substitutes for our senses 'see' with better and sharper vision than our eyes do, they hear finer nuances than our ears do, and they analyze each substance better than is possible for our tongues—though, partly, this is because our sense of taste has been dulled by the artificial flavorings in our food and, what is more, our noses have lost their keenness in learning to tolerate the chemical waste polluting the atmosphere. Since we no longer trust our senses, and are low on self-confidence, we are compelled to rely on technical equipment for picking up signals from the outside world, at the expense of a progressive blunting of these senses. This blunting (a species of self-protection against uncongenial work and incessant overstimulation) is supposed to be compensated for by technical aids—a false hope when an important quality is lost to us.

The more accurately we ascertain the dimensions of the universe, and the more dramatic our advances in measurement technology, the more one-sided do we become. Our material resources are almost unlimited, but we possess only a small fund of ideas. To be sure, we can measure, but our measurements are mere abstractions. Since the viewer watching ski racing cannot separate the leaders by a hundredth of a second, a five-figure digital timer is cut in on the TV screen to help. Then again, spectrum analysis can tell us the exact color of our eyes, but the result is hard for anyone to visualize.

Consequently, it may pay us to take an open-minded look at an alternative medical system, the product of an ancient foreign culture. Although contemporary Ayurveda does not in any way renounce the advances of modern science, it does place confidence in the subjective perceptions of our senses and in intuition. To an Ayurvedic physician, the flavor of a remedy is a clue to its power to correct some imbalance in the basic elements of being.

7

THE KEY OF LIFE
The Three Supporters

All matter is built on the basis of the *Mahabhutas*, or building blocks of existence, but only living matter has the *Tridoshas*, the three forces regulating all biological processes.* They arise out of the basic elements and are treated in Ayurvedic literature as substances although they are not. What they *are* is dynamic principles, three different forms of energy which govern the whole energy economy in living organisms. From the simplest activity in a cell to the most complicated of bodily functions, the *Tridoshas* permit and control everything that is going on. They always work as a team and one never appears without the others. Their interplay, their harmony or disharmony, decides the objective condition of a living being. A harmonious relationship of the three bioenergetic principles is the mark of good health. Any imbalance—and the equilibrium is very unstable—reveals itself in a wide variety of symptoms.

The *Tridoshas* (inner principles of the living body) are influenced by external factors, by sensory influences, and by foodstuffs. Therefore, Ayurvedic therapy can restore the physical balance of the three forces by means of 'nourishment' in the widest sense of the word.

The *Tridoshas* have acquired a specific character from the elements that rule them. The elements earth and water rule the formation of *Kapha*, fire rules that of *Pitta*, air and ether that of *Vata*. With a little practice, it is not difficult to recognize ways in which the *Tridoshas* express themselves. *Kapha* has the firmness and stability of earth, plus a fluid plasticity. *Pitta* displays the energy of fire, and *Vata* possesses the mobility of air and ether.

---

* Translator's note: According to some traditionalist Indian writers, these forces are known as *Dhatus*, or 'supporters,' when they are in normal healthy equilibrium and as *Doshas*, or 'faults,' only when unbalanced and unhealthy. The author of the present book has adopted a somewhat different view, confining the word *Dhatus* to its secondary meaning of 'tissues' and treating the *Doshas* as 'bioenergetic principles.'

The principle *Vata* is responsible for all the body's sensations and activities. Perception, assimilation, and reaction are all properties of *Vata*, which channels perceptions through the sense organs, transforms them into psychic events, and produces an appropriate reaction via the executive organs. *Vata* converts everything experienced by the senses into psychosomatic reactions, and so is often equated with vital force, or vitality; equating it with these does have something to be said in its favor, since *Vata* animates the psyche, regulates the breathing, and creates activity. In fact, it is the initiator and promoter of all biological action. Even the two other *Doshas* receive their motive energy from *Vata*.

The principle *Pitta* belongs to every reaction in which heat is generated. Its main function is all kinds of transformation of food in the body, all metabolic processes. *Pitta* has the energy of the element fire, and the nature of fire is to alter substances, to 'metamorphosize' combustible materials, to create warmth, and to be vivid and restless. *Pitta* is known as the impetus of life; it stimulates the intellect and the capacity for enthusiasm and encourages singleness of mind.

The principle *Kapha* is formative. It structures everything from individual cells to the skeletal frame; it lends strength and stability and also makes the body supple. Mental and physical strength and endurance, a well-knit frame, and putting on weight are all results of *Kapha*. This principle can accelerate the healing process and can build up resistance against disease. Generally speaking, wherever the effects of *Vata* and *Pitta* are seen in the body, *Kapha* keeps these two forces confined within their natural limits.

Sri Sivatatvaratnakara describes the different qualities of plants in terms of the ruling *Dosha* as follow: 'If a tree is tall and slender or if, on the other hand, it is stunted, if it shows signs of dryness or reduced sensitivity, if its blossoms and fruit are poorly formed, then it belongs to the *Vata* type. A tree that will not tolerate the blazing sun, a tree with a light-colored bark and pale leaves, bearing premature fruit and defective in the form and arrangement of its branches belongs to the *Pitta* type. A fully developed plant having a sturdy trunk and strong branches, bearing plenty of flowers and fruit, and with a spreading top and twining creepers belongs to the *Kapha* type.'

Lately, attempts have been made to find up-to-date medical equivalents for the traditional doctrine of the *Tridoshas*.[20] Thus it is postulated that *Vata* performs most of its functions through the release of acetylcholine both in the central brain and throughout the body at the endings of the parasympathetic nerves and in the peripheral nerves of the voluntary muscles. The functions of *Pitta* are equated with the activities of the sympathetic nervous system, which have mainly to do with energy discharge and catabolism. The action of *Kapha* is likened to that of the histamines, which regulate the fluid balance in the tissues and organs and increase the permeability of the capillaries for fluid exchange.

However, these definitions tell only part of the story and, even so, they are based on false analogies. The sole reason for proposing them is the desire to put Ayurveda on the same footing as industrialized medicine; but Ayurveda does not need such a dubious compliment. Admittedly, there are bound to be points of similarity between alternative medical systems, but their special contributions lie in the points where they differ. The distinctive quality of *Tridosha* doctrine is not that it is capable of being reinterpreted for Western consumption but that it explains energy processes in the organism.

The *Tridoshas* working in man determine, according to their relative strengths, the constitutional types and temperaments. They mold the basic character of individuals. People from each of the three psychosomatic character types differ from one another in state of health, in susceptibility to certain diseases, and in their response to medications (with allergic reactions, for example). They also differ in their emotions, in the way their minds work, and in their handling of external conditions.

This is where Ayurvedic diagnosis, which looks at the whole man, is able to score, based as it is on the *Tridoshas* and their disturbances. Therapy, too, is guided by the same condition of the *Doshas*.

It is necessary for the Ayurvedic physician to be able to recognize deviations from the norm in the *Tridosha* relationship and for him to know how to restore the balance by means of healing herbs, diet and mental or physical exercise. He has to find the cause of the loss of balance. This means taking into consideration the patient's environment with its physical and spiritual influences, 'for no event, no transaction, no word, no thought, no semblance or reality with which body or mind comes into contact, fails to exercise some influence however small on the *Tridoshas*.'[21]

In our machine-age medicine, the doctor endeavours to identify the disease from which the patient is suffering. 'The patient is downgraded into an object, a number, a diseased organ. Our medicine is the result of a purely materialistic world-view; in it are reflected the same problems we experience in our dealings with life, our fellow men and women, and nature.'[22] Yet mechanistic medicine is all right in its proper place. It is at its best in situations 'where man is all body'—in surgery, for example, when he has been rendered unconscious for a time, or in intensive care, where a detailed knowledge of how to link the human body to support systems is required. Generally speaking, then, scientific medicine with its allopathic (that is to say, predominantly synthetic) remedies suits situations in which the human 'architecture' has been damaged and must be repaired before it can start functioning properly again.[23]

Homeopathy, on the other hand, although its therapeutic means are very different from those employed by Ayurveda, has a very similar approach to people as patients, judging by the following statement: 'Homeopathy concerns itself in diagnosis and therapy with the physical, mental and spiritual planes in man, and thus with his inherited and acquired spiritual, mental and physical constitution and modes of reaction. This is the basis of individual possibilities for overcoming problems and conflicts, and also for dealing with illnesses. The patient as a spiritual being is not object, but subject.'[24]

Psychosomatic medicine, still something of a stepchild to our school medicine but coming increasingly into its own, could be a synthesis of the alternative medical systems—and I include Ayurveda among them—available in the Western world. No matter how much they differ among themselves, the important thing is for man to be seen once more as a unit and as a microcosm within the macrocosm.

8

THE POWER OF THE WIND

The Principle Known as Vata

Of the three forces, *Vata* is the most important, since it sets the two other *Doshas* in motion. Most of the functions ascribed to *Vata* in the classical texts have something to do with movement, with activity, with breathing, animation, and inspiration. Air and ether, the dominant elements in *Vata*, lend it their characteristics. Ether (*Akasha*) has the meaning of 'space;' air (*Vayu*) also means 'wind,' and the two meanings are combined in *Vata*, which is movement in space, in the microcosm, and in man.

As has already been mentioned, the *Tridoshas* form basic human character, and the dominant *Dosha* determines the psychosomatic character type to which an individual belongs. Of course, to talk of three types is an oversimplification, since we all belong to mixed types in which each of the three *Doshas* has some part to play. In this character typology based on old sources, subordinate effects are ignored and the dominant *Dosha* is taken as a general guide to a person's attitude and behaviour.

Similar guides have been worked out by the savants of all cultures and ages. Thus the *Vata* prototype in Ayurveda corresponds to the sanguine type of the ancient Greek physician and medical writer Galen, to the asthenic type of Kretschmer, and to the ectomorphs in Sheldon's typology. At the back of all these classifications lies the thought that, by providing ourselves with a few heavily stylized pictures as a yardstick, we shall find it to easier to make sense of the real-life impressions of those we wish to study.

In his book on the connection between Ayurveda and yoga, Dr. Rocque Lobo refers to the fundamental differences between the structures of Indian and Western thought. After placing the typology of Kretschmer side by side with the classical texts of the Vagbhata for purposes of comparison, he has this to say: 'Whereas Kretschmer lays great emphasis on physique, the writer of the Ayurvedic texts seems to have relied on sets of impressions—impressions that would be made on the observer by individuals of various types . . . It is as if the object of the Vagbhata were to make us reflect on our own behaviour towards our fellow men and women. In point of fact, an individual's character traits may be quite unlike what would be expected from his build according to Kretschmer's typology.'[25]

According to Vagbhata the *Vata* type is 'unstable in his decisions, in his dealings, in his discernment, in his friendships, in his opinions, and in his gait.' In other words, he is something of a weathercock. The description seems to have no redeeming features. We are told that people of this type have a reduced life expectancy, are lacking in energy and enthusiasm, and enjoy less sleep than normal. Their hair is thin, brittle, and lifeless. Their skin is rough and dry. Their voice tires easily and sounds cracked. They are hesitant and procrastinating, lack confidence, and hate the cold. These people like eating and prefer sweet, sour, pungent, and hot foods. They are tall and thin, and they walk noisily. Their gaze is penetrating and unfriendly. They are not popular with the opposite sex and have few offspring.

The unhappy individual described in these and in many other details is one we are never likely to meet, since in practice the pure *Vata* type is modified by the other *Doshas*. However, the following is a tabulation of the specific signs of the *Vata* type:

- The whole body is thin. (A portly individual is very unlikely to be of a pronounced *Vata* type. Excessive fat cannot arise from excessive *Vata*).
- The skin is dry. (This will be true of the skin all over the body; we are not talking here of patches of skin affected by external influences—as the hands, for instance, are affected by detergents.)
- The fingernails and toenails are rough and cracked and tend to be dark-colored (bluish or blackish). Nail biting is a typical symptom.
- The teeth are fragile; they are liable to plaque and dental decay.
- Sudden cramps are not unusual.
- Food is eaten in a rush; it is not chewed thoroughly and it often goes down the wrong way. Meal times are irregular, and the quantities consumed are irregular, too.
- The movements are restless and fitful (it is almost beyond the person's power to sit still). The eyes, too, are restless: they blink a lot, and the glance shifts rapidly from side to side. The joints crack.
- The sexual needs are not strong. The capacity for enjoyment is limited.
- The development of the intellect is erratic, and the memory is

unreliable. Concentration is generally weak.

- The whole life-style is marked by irregularities at every stage. There is a tendency to make hasty and ill-considered decisions. The individual has few friends and is often envious and dissatisfied.

The classical texts even go so far as to associate characteristic dream themes with the three prototypes. Thus, the *Vata* type often has dreams of flying and of climbing mountains and tall trees. Such dreams reflect an inclination to rise 'like smoke ascending from a joss-stick.'

The principle *Vata* takes from its constituent elements the properties it imparts to *Vata*-type individuals. It is:

- *ruksa*, dry, rough, abrasive.
- *sita*: cooling, cold.
- *laghu*: light.
- *suksma*: subtle, fine, penetrating.
- *sara*: movable, fluid.
- *visada*: clear, transparent, not viscous.
- *khara*: raw, loose.

Dry and cold are the two most active properties of *Vata*. They dominate. In conjunction with one or both of the other *Doshas*, *Vata* can have different effects: in conjunction with *Kapha* it is only cooling, because although *Kapha* is certainly cooling, it is also oily and fattening. In conjunction with *Pitta*, *Vata* can also be warming, since *Pitta* imparts heat. Now, because *Vata* is the initiator of movement in both the other *Doshas*, its effects extend into the areas covered by *Kapha* and *Pitta*. Hence it is possible that where there is an increase in *Kapha* or *Pitta* the real cause is some disturbance in *Vata*.

The classical Ayurvedic author, Susruta, describes *Vata* as the driving force that keeps everything going, but also as the main cause of disruption. Because *Vata* guides and controls the nerve processes involved in movement, in our emotions, in eating, in drinking, and in our general metabolism, its disturbances have far-reaching consequences.

Even a cursory examination will reveal when there is an excess of *Vata*: the skin is rough and appears dry and dark, and the frame is wasted; the individual suffers from tremors and has a strong desire for heat and hot things; he is a martyr to insomnia, has no strength, and his bowel movements are disordered. When *Vata* is deficient, the individual feels tired and exhausted, is asthmatic, ill-humored, and unable to concentrate.

The following is a comparative table of the features of a well-balanced *Vata* (physiological *Vata*) and of a disordered *Vata* (pathological *Vata*):

Vata

PHYSIOLOGICAL **Normal Function**	PATHOLOGICAL **Disturbed Function**
Proper regulation of all the body's activities.	The body's activities are impaired, upset, and inhibited.
Fitness for conception. Healthy development of the foetus. Natural parturition.	Fit for conception. Malformation or miscarriage of foetus. Uterine inertia.
Normal initiation of the movements for eating, digestion, and excretion.	The movements for eating, digestion, and excretion are disturbed or even paralyzed.
Mental activity. Control and guidance of mental processes.	Mental inactivity and confusion. Memory impaired.
Good control of the organs of perception and of the reactions of the executive organs.	The normal functions of perception and reaction are disturbed. Dulling of the senses and slowing of the responses.
Stimulation of digestion and of the secretion of gastric and other digestive juices.	Deficient secretion of gastric and other digestive juices.
Initiation of the wish and will to lead an active life. Imparts vitality and natural excitation.	Loss of energy and of the joy of living or else overexcitement.
Drying up of excessive and pathological discharges provoked by the two other *Doshas*.	Pathological discharges due to an unbalanced state of the other two *Doshas* are no longer dried up and combated.
Keeping the breathing regular.	Respiratory disorders.
Reinforcement of the life flow, promotion of longevity.	Obstruction of the life flow, shortening of life.

This diversity of functions—with its inherent risk of functional disorders—belongs to *Vata*, which is a general principle known as the 'power of the wind.' Ayurveda divides this general principle into five subsidiary forms, differing from one another by their localizations in the body and by their particular functions, although together they make up the 'power *Vata*'. They are *Prana, Udana, Vyana, Samana,* and *Apana.*[26]

The general localization of *Vata* as a whole is in the lower abdominal cavity and in the extremities, but the 'root' or *Vata* is in the colon. This is a very important fact for herbal therapy because, obviously, the colon is the field in which the main battle to eliminate any excess of *Vata* will have to be fought.

The chief sites of *Prana Vata* are the heart, head, and thorax, with further localizations in the brain, in the eyesight, in the ears, in the nose, and in the tongue. *Prana* means life. The leading functions of *Prana Vata* are to maintain the action of the heart and the functioning of the mental faculties of perception, understanding, and (especially) concentration; also to care for the arteries, veins, and nerves. To these we must add the auxiliary functions of inspiration, swallowing, expectoration, eructation, and sneezing.

The seat of *Udana Vata* is in the navel, in the lungs, and in the larynx. *Udana Vata* tends to rise and makes speech possible because it brings about the vibration of the vocal cords. Disturbed *Udana Vata* is especially evident in speech defects such as stuttering. Its other functions are preservation of physical strength and the fortification of intellect, memory, and understanding.

Vyana Vata transports nutrients and blood through the entire organism (circulatory disorders are disturbed *Vyana Vata*). Its main focus is the heart. *Vyana Vata* as a flowing force effects both the movement of the body and movement within the body. This is that aspect of *Vata which also moves the principles Pitta* and *Kapha. Vyana* represents the sum total of all the body's connections with the heart.

Samana Vata has its main focus around the navel and in the region of the stomach and small intestine. It is essential to normal digestion. Actually, the real work of digestion is done by the 'digestive fire' *Agni* and by *Pachaka Pitta*, but the 'power of the wind' *Samana Vata* fans the digestive fire into flame and keeps it burning. It selects useful substances from the chyme and supplies them to the body, and it aids the passage of waste products through the colon.

Apana Vata is focused in the rectum but occupies additional sites in the bladder and the genitals. It has a tendency to travel downward; it moves in the whole urinogenital tract and regulates defecation and urination, the menses, labor pains, and ejaculation.

There are many possible causes which might throw the principle

Vata out of equilibrium. For instance, an unbalanced diet can augment Vata. Wrong nourishment can be recognized by the sense of taste. Taste (Rasa), which will be studied in more detail in a later chapter, is our most natural instrument for determing whether or not we are eating the right things. As we learn to distinguish different types of taste, we begin to recognize the flavors of unhealthy food and chemical products.

Foods, and medicinal herbs with an unusually pungent, bitter, or astringent taste increase Vata. Examples are leguminous plants, hot spices, and even tea or coffee. All medicinal substances and food items having the above-mentioned tastes are drying and cooling; they are light, penetrating, and mobile, and loose but not sticky. All these properties of foodstuffs are also properties of Vata.

However, irregular meals, hunger, and vitamin B deficiency also intensify Vata, and the same effect is produced by physical overexertion or heavy work in a cold, raw, and dry climate. Outrageous and violent behavior will also agitate Vata.

In the Ayurvedic writings mention is made of certain times when individuals are especially prone to Vata disorders: the rainy season (monsoon), early morning before sunrise (the time between two and five AM), and early afternoon (roughly from two to five PM). An important part is also played by the time following the complete digestion of food, when the stomach is empty. Turning now to mental influences, we find that Vata is disturbed by anxiety, great grief, and excessive pleasurable sensations. The whole period of old age, from about sixty onward, is ruled by the Vata principle.

A disturbed and intensified Vata produces symptoms such as a rough skin and a look of emaciation. The entire appearance changes: the face loses its healthy color and seems generally darker. Every overstimulated Dosha is recognizable by a characteristic hue. The leading coloration of Vata is dark, bordering on black. Both skin and nails turn darker, and so do the urine and feces, which are hardened as well. Further symptoms are twitching, vertigo, constipation, and insomnia. Progressive weakening is also evident as is an increasing desire for hot water, hot food, and warmer clothing.

And so the Ayurvedic physician can recognize the typical signs of the person in whom Vata dominates; if not at first glance, then on closer observation. He sees the desiccated, enfeebled body; the light but uncertain steps; the unsteadiness in comportment, gestures and behavior; the restless limbs and eyes; he hears the rough, broken-sounding voice; notices the unusual talkativeness, the demandingness, and the readiness to take decisions without considering them carefully enough. This individual is easily irritated and is quick and unthinking in his likes and dislikes. Another noticeable trait is the speed with which he takes things in—and the speed with which he forgets them! The aversion to cold is typical, and the tendency to take a chill. All these observations point clearly to the dominance of *Vata*.

Frequently, the balance of power between the *Tridoshas* is not so clear-cut, and only some of the *Vata* characteristics can be recognized. Therefore the Ayurvedic physician begins with an eight-fold investigation (*Yogaratnakara*), and diagnoses certain partial aspects which should reveal the *Vata* influence with a reasonable degree of precision. When *Vata* dominates, the results of the eight diagnoses are more or less as follows:

- The pulse (*Nadi*) is rapid, thin, and 'like the movement of a snake.'
- The urine (*Mutra*) is frothy and has a dark brown color.
- The feces (*Malam*) are dry and hard and verging on black. The patient tends to be constipated.
- The tongue (*Jihva*) is dry and furrowed, its color ranging from bluish to blackish.
- The voice (*Shabda*) is dry, rough, and hoarse; the vocal cords are sore, and there is a dry cough.
- The skin (*Sparsa*) is dry, rough, cracked, and numb. The color turns dark; the skin feels cold.
- The eyes (*Drika*) lack moisture and do not shine. The pupils are contracted.
- The face, the overall impression (*Akriti*) is ash gray in color. The patient is fearful and does not fight the disease.

On the other hand, a reduction in *Vata* shows itself in the symptoms of the slowing down of all the body's activities, in fits of depression, in flabbiness of the limbs, and in reduced receptivity. The patient has difficulty in putting his words together fluently. These symptoms are similar to those caused by an increase in *Kapha*. A reduced *Vata* can be due to all those substances and factors that are employed in treating an increased *Vata*.

In the classical texts, eighty diseases or symptoms of disease are mentioned as being caused by an unbalanced state of *Vata*. The groups to which they belong are:

- All types of muscle and nerve pain. In general, there is no pain without the influence of *Vata*.
- Cramps and convulsions.

- Paralysis (from reduced *Vata*).
- All symptoms due to a vitamin B deficiency.

A good, regulating influence on this cold, dry, rough *Vata* is exerted by heat and oil therapies and by inhalations and massage. In cases of weakness, food and medicinal herbs tasting salty, sweet, and sour are calming and strengthening when given internally. Items with these tastes are heating and lubricating and help the body to put on weight. Their most important properties are coarseness, stability, gelatiousness, and smoothness. With the help of these properties of the *Gunas* they are soothing and smoothing. Examples of such food items are grain, fruit, milk, and meat broth.

Rest and relaxation are simple therapeutic measures for calming *Vata*. As therapy for a weakened *Vata* we can use everything that has the same properties as *Vata*; that is to say, those factors that we have named as *Vata* strengtheners. In an acute illness, provided the patient is not too weak, the patient is always cleansed of any excess of *Doshas* before anything else is attempted. *Vata* is eliminated by means of an oil enema combined with a plant extract, the idea being to deal with the root of the disturbed *Vata* (i.e., in the colon) and then the disturbed *Vata* in the upper body will settle down. This is because, when the roots of a tree are cut, the leaves and blossoms also die, as do the shoots and fruit, the trunk and branches.'

9

THE POWER OF FIRE
The Principle Known as Pitta

The principle known as *Pitta* is the energy released by chemical and biochemical processes. Its main carriers in the body are the hormones, enzymes, and coenzymes. Its activities are similar to the functions of the sympathetic nervous system, which are concerned mainly with the breaking down of complex molecules in the body and with the liberation of energy (catabolism).

In the classical texts, the most important functions of this power of the inner fire are given as digestion, combustion, metabolic transformation, oxidation, visual faculty, regulation of the body temperature, and the color of the blood and skin. The normal appearance and ambience of a person depend on *Pitta*.

The effects of this life principle on the mind are chiefly to produce intelligence, a sound memory, enthusiasm that can border on ecstasy, a lively awareness, boldness, and high ideals.

In its pure form *Pita* would bestow on an individual the following chracteristics:

- A body possessing little strength or resistance. Limited ability to sustain physical exertion (the person would be no marathon runner). Loose joints, flabby muscles, and warm limbs. Good circulation in the hands and feet.
- Light yellowish or (quite often) reddish skin. Moles, freckles, and birthmarks. Palms, soles, lips, and tongue that are redder than in the other types. Small, active eyes with fine but scanty lashes.
- Slow-growing hair which easily falls out and turns gray early.
- A liking for eating too much and too often and for punctual meals (the individual often carries a snack in his pocket to 'tide him over'). The need to drink a lot. A preference for cold or chilled food in the following taste range: sweet (*madhura*), bitter (*tikta*), and astringent (*kasaya*). The excretion of urine and feces is very abundant, and there is a tendency to diarrhea.

- The *Pitta* type often likes to use perfumes and deodorants, since he perspires freely.
- Moderate sexual desires, no great sex appeal, and limited popularity with the opposite sex.
- Great intelligence, a good memory, and logical thought. Rapid decision-making and consistency in the handling of affairs. What is said is clear and to the point and is often sharp and aggressive. Quick temper and liable to be very jealous. A latent belligerence. Possibility of considerable vindictiveness and aptness to be judgmental; on the other hand, willingness to experiment, much initiative, and a sense of responsibility.

The classical texts of the *Vagbhata* also describe the symbols recurring in this person's dreams: meteors, bright horizons, lightning flashes, fire, and the sun. His dream plants are 'sharp' in nature.

The *Pitta* prototype is similar in its typology to the choleric of Galen, the athletic of Kretschmer, and the mesomorph of Sheldon.

The fundamental properties of fire, its element of origin, are shared by the life principle *Pitta*, and are manifested as:

- *usna* (hot)
- *tiksna* (sharp)
- *drava* (fluid)
- *sara* (mobile)

and to a lesser extent
- *snigdha* (oily, viscous)

A further property of *Pitta* is the occurrence of all colors with the exception of white. A fishy smell is another sign of *Pitta*.

Some of the obvious indications when *Pitta* is disturbed are an ill appearance, yellow or red skin color, reduced skin absorbency, anxiety, and irritation.

The following table highlights the differences between a balanced and an unbalanced *Pitta*:

Pitta

PHYSIOLOGICAL **Normal Function**	PATHOLOGICAL **Disturbed function**
Activation and regulation of the digestion.	Poor digestion. Imperfect separation of nutrients and waste materials.

Preserves the vision.	Impaired vision.
Regulates body temperature.	Body temperature irregular.
Definite skin color. Normal appearance and impression.	Ill appearance. Various skin colors.
Courage.	Anxiety.
A happy disposition.	Irritability dominates.
Colors the blood.	A deficiency of hemoglobin.
Promotes intellectual capacity.	Mental apathy. Deficient intelligence.
Absorbs substances smeared on the skin.	Reduced absorbency of the skin.
High ideals. A striving for real values.	Spiritual poverty.

The 'Power of Fire,' like the 'Power of the Wind,' is divided into five varieties. The 'five fires,' *Alochaka, Pachaka, Ranjaka, Sadaka, and Bhrajaka*, taken together represent the force known as *Pitta*.[27] The main site of Pitta as a whole is the lower thorax or upper abdomen. For therapy with medicinal herbs it its important to remember the location of the 'root of *Pitta*' in the small intestine.

The main site of *Alochaka Pitta* is the eyes, and it causes the faculty of sight.

Pachaka Pitta, 'the fire of digestion,' is located between the stomach and the duodenum. Its function is the biological process of digestion and combustion. *Pachaka Pitta* separates what is usable in food from what is unusable, and brings about the production of hydrochloric acid in the stomach. A sharpened appetite and a craving for specific substances come from *Pachaka Pitta*.

Ranjaka Pitta is the 'coloring fire.' It is formed in the liver, and its field of action is the stomach, liver, and spleen. Its main site is the stomach, where it is clearly felt when there is any sudden stress. *Ranjaka Pitta* is also known as 'fighting fire' or 'aggressive fire.' Comparable expressions are current in our own language: 'I see red!' or 'I am flaming mad!,' 'burning anger,' or 'a fiery fighter.' If *Ranjaka Pita* is obstructed, it seizes the stomach itself and causes gastric ulcers. It warms the life-fluid and colors it red.

Sadhaka Pitta is the 'fire of the heart.' The heart is regarded as the seat of consciousness. The functions of *Sadhaka Pitta* have therefore to do with the mind and soul—intelligence, memory, clear thinking, emotions, self-reliance, and the capacity for enthusiasm—and all depend on a balanced *Sadhaka Pitta*.

Bhrajaka Pitta is the 'fire that makes radiant' and its main location is the entire surface of the skin. Whether or not a person is glowing with health is determined by this fire. If a person is 'looking radiant,' then that person's *Bhrajaka Pitta* is harmonious. Another interesting point is that this fire's effects reach deep into the psyche, because it is generally responsible for our inner reactions to outside impressions and for our ability to give and take when communicating with others.

Pitta strengtheners include, first and foremost, foods and medicines which are sour, salty, and pungent, for example, strong-flavored meals containing too much chili, pepper, or nutmeg, too much acid fruit or sour milk or yoghurt. Basically, these foods are heating and penetrating; they are also fluid and movable. They increase the metabolic rate, strengthen the circulation of the blood, and stimulate the functioning of the glands.

Fierce heat and overexposure to the sun will also augment *Pitta*.

In the psyche, it is feelings such as aggravation, grief, fear, and rage which bring an upsurge of *Pitta*.

The times of the year and day when *Pitta* is liable to be disordered are summer (the dry season in the tropics), the middle of the day (between ten AM and two PM), and the middle of the night (between ten PM and two AM). The period during which meals are being digested is also unfavorable as far as *Pitta* is concerned.

Middle life, between the ages of thirty and sixty, is dominated by the principle *Pitta*. An overstimulated and augmented *Pitta* expresses itself in quite distinctive symptoms such as yellowing of the skin, the whites of the eyes, the feces, and the urine; by a high temperature and fever; by a craving for cold food and drink; by insomnia, general weakness, and reduced perception through the senses (especially the eyesight); and by thirst, a sensation of burning, and vertigo. Also, all signs of inflammation, suppuration, and gangrene are symptoms of unbalanced *Pitta*.

The dominance of the principle *Pitta* in an individual may be recognized by typical characteristics. Hotness (*usna*) in *Pitta* causes an intolerance of hot things; gives sensations of hunger and thirst; and produces moles, birthmarks, premature wrinkles, and graying of the hair. The property pungent (*tiksna*) gives a strong digestion with a love of eating and drinking, but also the inability to meet difficult situations effectively. From the property fluid (*drava*) come elasticity and flexibility of the muscles and tendons, as well as profuse perspiration and increased excretion of urine and feces.

Yogaratnakara, the eightfold method of diagnosis, permits us to recognize various infallible signs of an increase in *Pitta*:

- The pulse (*Nadi*) is full and is more rapid than usual or 'like a jumping frog.'
- The urine (*Mutra*) is clear and hot. It is a yellow to reddish color (due to pigments of blood and bile), and there is a scalding sensation when urinating.
- The feces (*Malam*) are loose to watery and are yellow or blood-stained.
- The tongue (*Jihva*) is red and swollen.
- The voice (*Shabda*) sounds 'heated' and angry and the words tend to tumble out. There is an impulse to try and convince others by shouting at them.
- The skin (*Sparsa*) is soft and looks smooth, red-coloured, and shining. Yellow and red patches. Increased perspiration.
- The eyes (*Drika*) exhibit defective vision, red venules, inflammation of the eyes, and yellow whites.
- The face (*Akriti*) gives the general impression of restlessness, anxiety, and apprehension. Exaggerated emotions. The patient tries to fight the illness.

A reduced and weakened *Pitta* is revealed in an obvious loss of body heat, a poor appetite, and a loss of the normal healthy glow.

A reduced *Pitta* can be due to all those factors that are employed in treating an increased *Pitta*.

In the classical texts, forty diseases or symptoms (as the case may be) are mentioned as being caused by an unbalanced *Pitta*. The basic disease groups are as follows:

- Gastro-enterological disorders caused by disturbed *Pachaka Pitta*. The symptoms are deficient digestion, increased production of gastric juice, heartburn, gastritis, stomach ulcer, relutance to eat.
- Disorders which show themselves in the secretions. The symptoms are heavy perspiration, unpleasant body odor, hot, scalding, or red-stained urine and feces.
- Inflammations, infections.
- Liver function disorders.
- Clouded, impaired vision.
- Diseases in which red and yellow colors appear.

The classic Ayurvedic texts also mention graying of the hair, irritation, and despondency as *Pitta* disorders.

The treatment of increased *Pitta* is initially by diet and medicinal herbs tasting bitter, sweet, and astringent. Foods having these tastes are cooling, mollifying, solidifying, and stabilizing. Astringent drugs are those containing tannin, such as oak bark, sage, or blackberry leaves, and these therefore stabilize and contract the mucous membranes. Examples of sweet substances are sugarcane juice and coconut milk, which help when the liver function is upset. Cool, pleasant, and stress-free surroundings will, of course, make the therapy more effective.

When *Pitta* is weak, all those factors should be employed which have the same properties as *Pitta* and will therefore help to strengthen it.

In the classical texts, a cleansing therapy is recommended as the initial treatment when *Pitta* is overly strong—provided the patient is not too debilitated, of course. Expectant mothers and children are also excepted from the treatment.

Since the root of *Pitta* lies in the small intestine, laxatives are the appropriate cleansers. As has been said: 'A hot oven cools down once the fire inside has been raked out.'

10

THE POWER OF COHESION
The Principle Known as Kapha

Without the power of *Kapha*, the material universe would be as formless as wind and fire and would have no cohesion. The basic elements of which it is composed are earth and water, which, when mixed, give mud and clay. In the earliest scriptures, we are told that mankind was formed from clay.* Generally speaking, clay was the first plastic material to be discovered by man.

Where Genesis, the first book in the Bible, describes the creation of the elements followed by the formation of living things, many Europeans tend to see nothing but legends; to an Indian, however, the sequence of events recorded is perfectly logical. From the *Mahabhutas*, which are the foundation of existence, has been formed substance as well as every force that energizes organic matter from within. Earth and water are the building blocks of the force *Kapha*, an old Sanskrit name for which is *Slesma*, meaning 'cementing' or 'cohering.' And, in keeping with the properties of its components, *Kapha* imparts to the body stability, firmness, flexibility, resilience, and coolness.

The *Kapha* principle is involved in the construction of the smallest cell and of the largest bone in the body and in the formation of the joints, as well as in mental strength and endurance and in resistance to disease. These are its most important effects—to which we must add

* *Translator's note:* Formavit igitur Dominus Deus hominem de limo terrae, et inspiravit in faciem ejus spiraculum vitae, et factus est homo in animam viventem. 'And the Lord God formed man of the dust of the ground, and breathed into his nostrils the breath of life; and man became a living soul.' (Genesis, 2.7)

Ex hac illius conjunctione prodiit Mot; Id quod limum nonnulli, alii aqosae mixtionis corruptionem esse volunt ex qua sequutae productionis semina, ipsaque ado rerum universarum generatio extiterit. '. . . and of this, with that wind, was begotten Môt which some call Mud others the putrefaction of a watery mixture. And of this came all the seed of this building and the generation of the universe.' (Sanchoniatho the Phoenician in Eusebius, Praep. Evang. 1.10)

See also Apollodorus 'The Library' I.7.2.

its ability to accelerate the healing processes. One essential function of *Kapha* is to ensure the permeability of the cells. Intra- and extracellular fluids transport *Kapha* through the whole body. *Kapha* aids anabolism and so builds up the tissues.

The classical *Vagabhata* tests rhapsodize over the *Kapha* prototype with his sleek skin, supple muscles, broad, strong chest, lean limbs, good-looking, regular features, and his fertility and abundant vitality, passion and sensibility—sounding more like a hymn of praise than a sober description. Persons of this type are said to have the 'gait of a rutting elephant,' and a wide mental horizon, and are liable to dream of 'immense lakes with lotus flowers and swans,' or of 'flocks of birds and clouds.'

Nevertheless, in spite of this panegyric, it has to be remembered that the three forces are neither good nor bad in themselves but are positive when in harmony and negative when in disharmony; each individual belongs to some mixed type involving all three of the *Doshas*.

To sum up, the *Kapha* characteristics are as follows:

- Good physical stability guaranteeing endurance, strength, and staying power. Well-proportioned limbs and strong bones and muscles. (The *Kapha* type avoids inessential movements, generally prefers to take things steadily, and is content just to sit quietly.)
- The skin is greasy, soft, and shiny, is not very sensitive, and feels rather cool. The body tissues are well-developed, and the skin is correspondingly elastic.
- The hair is thick and slightly greasy. Its color is distinctive and strong.
- The individual eats slowly, and his digestion is excellent. He does not set undue store by punctual meal times. Food assimilation is extremely good, therefore, relatively small quantities of food are required in proportion to body size and strength.
- The aptitude for sexual activity is great, and there is a corresponding capacity for sensual enjoyment.
- The intelligence is as well-developed as in the *Pitta* type but takes more time to reach conclusions, which are, however, well thought out. The enunciation is clear and deliberate, and the voice is pleasant sounding.
- Life expectancy is good. The sleep requirement is not great. The individual is not easily upset or irritated.

Counterparts of *Kapha* in other typologies are the phlegmatic type (Galen), the pyknic (Kretschmer), and the endomorph (Sheldon).

Kapha, the forming and preserving power, owes its properties to the elements earth and water, and is: heavy (*guru*), oily (*snigdha*), turbid and gelatinous (*picchila*), cold (*sita*), coarse (*sthula*), stable (*sthira*), and smooth (*slaksma*). Other characteristics are the sweet taste (*madhura*) and the color white.

In general, *Kapha* appears where the effects of *Vata* and *Pitta* make themselves felt, and keeps the other two *Doshas* within their natural bounds. In the stomach, for example, *Kapha* will bring about the production of mucus to counteract an excess of hydrochloric acid caused by *Pitta*.

An increased and unbalanced *Kapha* is noticeable by pallor, excessive coldness, callosity, clamminess, dullness, slow reactions, itching, constipation, and a sweetish taste.

The following table lists the properties of harmonious and inharmonious *Kapha*:

Kapha

PHYSIOLOGY **Normal Function**	PATHOLOGY **Disturbed Function**
Moistens and lubricates.	Asynovia, and under-production of mucus in the digestive tract and of saliva.
Firmness of the joints.	Loose joints.
Hardness, stability, and compactness.	Softness, instability, and porosity.
Strength of character and determination.	Vacillation, weakness, and laziness.
Seriousness of intent.	Giving in easily.
Plumpness, firm muscle tone, and good state of nutrition.	Emaciation, poor state of nutrition.
Sexual potency.	Impotence.
Physical strength.	Physical weakness.
Willingness to forgive.	Revengefulness. Intolerance. Discontent.
Freedom from envy.	Envy and jealousy.

The many operations of the force *Kapha*, which extend from the body's most important functions far into the mental and character-building regions, occur (like those of the other *Doshas*) in five varieties: *Avalambka, Kledaka, Bodhaka, Tarpaka,* and *Slesaka*.[28] They differ in their locations and functions, but together they comprise the force *Kapha.*

In a general sense, the site of *Kapha* is the upper thoracic cavity, the stomach, and the head. Its 'root' is in the stomach, and that is where therapy with medicinal plants is applied.

Avalambaka Kapha is localized mainly in the region of the thorax and pelvis. In particular, it strengthens the heart, the sacrum, and the throat and is the most important manifestation of the *Kapha* principle for, without it, it would not be possible to keep *Sadhaka Pitta* viable, and then the heart would stop and the individual would die. *Avalambaka Kapha* also provides for the flexibility of the whole body and in the mental realm encourages the desire to keep busy but simultaneously holds the activity in check.

The word *avalambaka* means 'supportive.' According to the classical texts, this subprinciple maintains the four other *Kaphas* by supplying them with 'nutriment' via the *Vata* pathways. This ancient theory, based on observation, is borne out by the objective findings of modern medicine: The flexibility of the joints and limbs depends on the blood supply to the extremities of the body.

Kledaka Kapha moistens the food in the stomach and counteracts the fire of *Sadaka pitta.* The word *kledaka* means 'humidifying.' Its main site is in the stomach and in the duodenum. The internal 'lubrication' of the digestive organs, the function of moistening, corresponds to the release of a series of juices to mix with the ingested food. When the function is normal, there is a feeling of repletion and rest in the abdominal region; when it is below normal there is a sensation of inner emptiness.

Bodhaka Kapha makes taste possible. Its main location is in the mouth, the root of the tongue, and the throat. It regulates the flow of saliva and gives the ability to make fine differentiations and recognize nuances of flavor. When the mouth 'waters' that is the work of *Bodhaka Kapha,* and so is the so-called 'bitter taste left in the mouth' after encounters with certain people.

Tarpaka Kapha, in the head, nourishes, oils, and supports all the functions of the brain and sense organs, and regulates fluid exchange in the brain and the functions of *Prana Vata* and *Alochaka Pitta.*

Slesaka Kapha oils and lubricates the joints and makes them flexible. It also strengthens the ligaments.

What are the influences that reinforce *Kapha*? All sweet, sour, and salty foodstuffs and medicinal plants. It promotes weight increase and is fattening and cooling; in addition, it is gelatinous, coarse, static, and smooth. Examples of such foodstuffs are fats, carbohydrates, and an excess of sugar or salt. In general, overeating will bring about an increase in *Kapha*, and so will any snack taken before the previous meal has been digested. Too much sleep, especially sleep taken during the day, sedentary habits, and deficient physical and mental activity all work in the same direction.

Times of special risk for *Kapha* are spring, morning (between the hours of six and ten AM), early evening (between the hours of six and ten PM, and just after meals.

Childhood and youth are ruled by *Kapha*.

An intensification of and increase in *Kapha* are shown by a whitening of the skin, nails, and eyes. The feces and urine are pale as well. Other symptoms are shivering, sluggishness and faintness or exhaustion, deep sleep, stiff joints, an increased flow of saliva (dribbling), coughing, and respiratory disorders. In addition, there is a loss of appetite and a revulsion from food. At the main sites of *Kapha* there are white colorations, chilliness, itching, swelling, stiffness, loss of sensitivity, wetness, and sweetness. A marked psychological symptom is avarice or greed.

Yogaratnakara, the eightfold diagnostic method Ayurveda can detect the following clear-cut signs:

- The pulse (*Nadi*) is slow and regular, 'like a swan swimming in a pool' or like a dove, because its beat has no 'attack.'
- The urine (*Mutra*) is pale and turbid, due to undissolved albumin held in suspension.
- The feces (*Malam*) are pale, slimy to loose, and cause irritation.
- The tongue (*Jihva*) is furred (white) and swollen.
- The voice (*Shabda*) is low, soft, and sweet.
- The skin (*Sparsa*) is cold, white, greasy, and plump.
- The eyes (*Drika*): are clear, the whites are particularly white-looking, and the pupils are large.
- The face and general impression (*Akriti*) show unconcern, apathy, and self-pity.

A deficiency of *Kapha*, on the other hand, gives a rough skin, a rise of temperature, weakness in the joints, thirst, general debility, insomnia, and a sinking feeling.

In the classical texts, twenty diseases are mentioned which are caused by a disordered *Kapha*. These can be classified as follows:

- Respiratory disorders.
- Increased production of urine, feces, and saliva.
- Digestive disorders.
- Poor metabolism (diabetes).
- Reduced mental capacity (feeblemindedness).
- Weakness, lethargy.
- Sudden changes of taste.

To counteract an excess of *Kapha* medicinal plants and foods which are pungent, bitter, and astringent are used, owing to the fact that their properties are intensifying, heating, and drying. Examples of these are garlic, pepper, ginger, mustard seed, and plants containing volatile oils.

The usual treatment is a sweat cure, ideally with plenty of movement (possibly in a rubber sweatsuit to induce free perspiration). Psychologically important for the success of the therapy is a readiness to undertake exertion.

All the things that promote and increase *Vata* and *Pitta* reduce *Kapha*.

The first step to be taken when there is a superfluity of *Kapha* is that of cleansing to remove the dammed-up *Kapha*. For this purpose, the ancient texts recommend emetics, since the root of *Kapha* lies in the stomach. In other words, 'Just as the breaching of a dam prematurely withers the rice, an excess of *Kapha* will dry up when the surplus is ejected.'

11

THE RESTORATION OF HARMONY
A Casebook Example

Many diseases arise, not simply through one unbalanced *Dosha*, but through an imbalance in two or in all three of the *Doshas*. Thus, where one *Dosha* is strongly augmented, another may be weakly augmented, and the third may be reduced. Any combination is possible. For instance, if pain is being caused by suppuration, it is firstly *Pitta* that will be found to be strengthened and secondly *Vata*. In a typical *Kapha* complaint, such as obesity, *Pitta* is usually reduced, whereas *Kapha* is markedly increased.

I think that a practical example will best illustrate these interconnections. The basis of what follows comes from a lecture delivered by Prof. S. N. Tripathi at the University of Benares, showing the relationship of the *Tridoshas* to a given disease, the diagnosis, treatment, and cure of which reveals the light in which it is seen by contemporary Ayurveda.

The disease in question is *Tamaka's Swasa*. The term *Swasa* means dyspnoea, or difficult breathing. In the classical Ayurvedic texts, five different *Swasas* are mentioned, *Tamaka's Swasa* being the equivalent of what we now know as bronchial asthma.

The phenomena of bronchial asthma are, first, labored respiration and, second, a reduction in the ventilation necessary for gas exchange in the bronchi. Ventilation is reduced by two factors, one of which is a spasmodic contraction (due to increased *Vata*) and the other a swelling of the mucous membranes, with attendant secretion of tenacious mucus (due to increased *Kapha*). On the theory of the *Tridoshas*, Kapha in this disease is increased threefold, *Vata* is increased twofold, and *Pitta* is decreased onefold.

The affected *Srotas*—i.e., channels or transport routes in the body—are the *Prana Vaha Srotas* and the *Anna Vaha Srotas*. The *Prana Vaha Srotas* are the routes for respired air; they conduct the stream of oxygen to the blood. The *Anna Vaha Srotas* are the transport routes for solid and liquid nourishment. Now, lungs and stomach are closely connected on a number of levels:

- Embryonal: the lungs and stomach develop from the same germ layer.
- Pharmacological: certain medications will act either on the stomach or on the lungs according to the dosage—in weak doses acting as expectorants and in strong doses acting as emetics.
- Pathological: bronchial asthma is associated with deficient hydrochloric acid production in the stomach.
- Clinical: after the ingestion of food, there is an increase in *Kapha*, and this leads to an intensification of the symptoms of bronchial asthma.
- Therapeutic: vomiting helps to relieve bronchial asthma.

It is now time to take a look at the character type to which the patient belongs, and at how it affects his chances of recovery. In the *Kapha* type, a cure is particularly difficult to manage, and treatment takes a long time. Even in the *Vata* type, the chances are not optimal, treatment is complicated, and there are likely to be relapses. The *Pitta* type has the best chance of a cure; it is relatively easy to treat and recuperation is swift.

The basic treatment relies on the following measures:

- Antiallergy remedies and expectorants to reduce *Kapha*.
- Antispasmodic remedies to reduce *Vata*.
- Remedies aiding digestion that are designed to increase *Pitta*.
- Remedies that ease the breathing and are designed to increase *Pitta* and reduce *Vata*.
- Emetics and aperients as cleansers.

The attempt to restore harmony combines two approaches:

1 *Treatment directed at the 'Tridoshas'*:
   This is designed to strengthen the psyche and the organism as a whole, so that the body will be encouraged to throw off the disease.
      The means employed are those which reduce *Kapha* and *Vata* and strengthen *Pitta*. Medicinal plants with a pungent taste reduce *Kapha* and *Vata* and strengthen *Pitta*. Medicinal plants which are fundamentally fatty and oily and have a heating, therapeutic action reduce *Kapha* and *Vata*. Medicinal plants of which the transformed mode of action after digestion is 'pungent' strengthen *Pitta*. Examples of herbs which are effective in this last case are the peppers, black pepper and long pepper. Their taste (*Rasa*) is pungent, their basic qualities (*Gunas*) are fatness and hotness, their

medicinal action (*Virya*) is heating, and their transformed 'flavor' or mode of action after digestion (*Vipaka*) is also pungent.

2   *Disease-oriented treatment:*
    Here, plants are used which act on specific organs, thus having a powerful local effect. In this case, the pharmacological action (*Prabhava*) of the thorn apple is employed, since it relieves bronchospasm (cramplike contractions of the bronchial tubes).

These are the main principles governing the choice and compounding of medicinal plants, about which we shall say more later.

12

THE INTERIOR OF THE BODY
Tissues, Vessels, and Secretions

According to the classical definition of Charaka, an individual may be regarded as healthy only 'when the *Tridoshas* are in equilibrium, the seven *Dhatus* are normal, *Agni* is functioning properly, the thirteen large *Srotas* and the innumerable small ones are open, and the three *Malas* are correctly balanced.' The *Dhatus* are the fundamental tissues of the body, *Agni* is the fire of digestion (and so important that we are devoting the whole of the next chapter to it), the *Srotas* are the body's vessels or ducts, and the *Malas* are its wasteproducts.

The Ayurvedic physician relies on the keenness of his senses when he wants to appraise the leading properties of a medication. He recognizes the quality of an item of food and of a medicinal plant or drug by his sense of taste. The effect of the different flavors on the *Tridoshas*, and consequently on the tissues, vessels, and waste products, belong to the basics of medical knowledge; armed with these one can detect the therapeutic value of any fruit, herbs, drug, or article of diet.

The astringent taste (*Kasaya*), for instance, has an action on the *Tridoshas* that strengthens *Vata* and tones down *Pitta* and *Kapha*. This taste has a catabolic action on the tissue and helps to break them down so that they are ready for absorption, etc. Its action on the waste products is obstructing (e.g., constipating), antidiuretic, and flatulent. It has only a slight action on the vessels.

The *Dhatus* are the fundamental tissues of the body. They are formed from and nourished by *Ahara Rasa* (the so-called chyle, a milky juice found in the stomach and in the lymph vessels of the intestines). Progressive change between the tissues is the outcome of complex and involved metabolic processes in the microscopic region. On the basis of scientific knowledge gleaned over some thousands of years, Ayurvedic medicine has managed to trace subtle physiological relationships.

The seven fundamental tissues are *Rasa, Rakta, Mamsa, Meda, Asthi, Majja,* and *Sukra*. In these, various substances are converted into one another, and usable materials are separated from the refuse.

The predominant element of *Rasa Dhatu* is *Ap*, or water. *Rasa* corresponds to blood plasma, to parenchymatous fluid, and to lymph, converting solids into fluids and distributing them throughout the body.

Ingested food undergoes complicated processes removing it more and more from its original form and increasingly into something like the body's own substance. Chyle makes its appearance in an intermediate material called *Ahara Rasa*, which is neither food nor body tissue. This *Ahara Rasa* is changed into *Rasa Dhatu* with the help of *Agni*, the powerful principle of digestive fire. Hence *Rasa Dhatu* is a product of the process of digestion and with the help of *Vata* circulates through the whole body, nourishing every cell.

Like a Roman fountain pouring out water that splashes from one basin into the next below, so *Rasa Dhatu* supplies the other six *Dhatus* with essence. If this were not a permanent arrangement, we could say that the other Dhatus exist only from and through *Rasa Dhatu*.

The quality of *Rasa Dhatu* in a person may be judged by the condition of his skin. If *Rasa* is in a normal, healthy state, the skin is smooth and glistening, soft and delicate, and is covered by fine, deep-rooted hairs. There is a definite mental and physical 'glow'. Good health, vital force, joy, and a lively mind (and therefore not simply 'luck') are the signs of a healthy *Rasa Dhatu*.

When the *Dhatus* are thrown out of balance, it is because the *Doshas* are inharmonious. If *Rasa Dhatu* is much augmented by inharmonious *Doshas*, the result is nausea, a greater flow of saliva, and symptoms of increased *Kapha*. A reduction in *Rasa Dhatu* gives symptoms of cardiac palpitation, pains, hypersensitivity to noise, deafness, emaciation, debility, thirst, rough skin, and a feeling of oppression. The slightest effort is a strain.

The leading element in *Rakta Dhatu* is *Tejas*, or fire. *Rakta* corresponds to the blood constituents. Many sources say that *Rakta* 'is' the blood. Its function is to preserve life and to nourish the whole body. Today, it is standard practice all over the world to analyze the hemoglobin content of the blood, but the traditional method of physical examination is still useful. To see whether or not the blood constituents are in good order, take a look at the patient's ears, tongue, and oral cavity, lips, hands, soles of the feet, nails, and genitals, all of which should be reddish and well-shaped. The face, too, ought to have a healthy color. Psychologically, there should be cheerfulness, delicacy of feeling, and obvious intelligence. Heat and problems are borne only with difficulty, however.

Increased *Rakta* may be recognized by a red coloration of the eyes, skin, and urine. An obvious symptom is swollen blood vessels, giving rise to certain typical diseases such as spleen disorders, skin complaints, abscesses, gout, jaundice, hemorrhages, upset digestion, and coma.

Reduced *Rakta* may be recognized by rough, dry, and cracked skin and a feeling of bloodlessness. A craving for cold and sour food is typical.

The prevailing element of *Mamsa Dhatu* is *Prthivi*, or earth. *Mamsa* corresponds to muscle tissue and is responsible for muscular form and energy. *Mamsa Dhatu* is derived from *Rasa* and *Rakta*, and its most important function is to maintain *Meda Dhatu*.

Well-developed muscles reveal themselves at the temples, on the forehead, on the nape of the neck, around the eyes, in the cheeks, along the jaw, and in shoulders, abdomen, chest, arms, legs, over the pelvis, and at the joints of the hands and feet. But size is not a true criterion of muscle quality; the important thing is tensile strength. Psychological signs of a healthy condition of *Mamsa Dhatu* are patience, perseverance, stability, openness, health, and a feeling of strength and vitality.

Increased *Mamsa Dhatu* is apparent in increased fatty tissue and in a feeling of heaviness. The cheeks, lips, upper thighs, calves, abdomen, and penis are plump. Typical diseases are swellings in the region of the neck and also small- to medium-sized tumors. Reduced *Mamsa Dhatu* shows itself in wasting of the muscular and fatty tissues of the neck, abdomen, cheeks, lips, penis, upper thighs, calves, armpits, breasts, and around the eyes. Pinching pains and sore joints are quite usual.

Meda Dhatu has *Ap*, or *water*, and *Prthivi*, or *earth*, as its leading elements. It corresponds to the fatty tissue in the human body. Fatty tissue is maintained and nourished by *Mamsa Dhatu* (and in a wider sense through *Rasa*, *Rakta*, and *Mamsa*) and in its turn supports and forms *Asthi Dhatu*.

Meda is responsible for the lubrication of the body; it causes sudoration and a greasy appearance of the skin. When the elements of the fatty tissue are in good condition, the fact is apparent in the general elasticity of the body. The skin looks oily and feels pliable, the joints are supple and do not click. Even the voice sounds smooth. In the psychological realm there is frankness and healthful vitality and a spirit of friendliness to others.

The signs of increased *Meda Dhatu* are fattiness, putting on weight around the middle, and a rounding out of the breasts, as well as coughing and weakness. Reduced *Meda Dhatu* brings joint pains, dryness of the eyes, atrophy of the abdominal muscles, emaciation, and debility. A telltale sign is a generally gross build with weak joints. A liking for fatty foods is typical. Diseases involving spleenic tumors are also due to a reduced *Meda Dhatu*.

The basic elements of *Asthi Dhatu* are *Prthivi* and *Vayu*, or earth and air. This shows us what to expect, for bones and bone tissue (as indicated by the blend of earth and air in *Asthi Dhatu*) must be strong but porous—if they were not full of hollows they would be much too heavy.

A healthy, normal condition of *Asthi Dhatu* reveals itself in strong, prominent joints and knuckles, a firm chin and bony skull, and strong bones, nails, and teeth. Psychologically, a healthy *Asthi Dhatu* spells enthusiasm and activity and the ability to face great hardships.

An overemphasized *Asthi Dhatu* gives enlarged bones and teeth. On the other hand, when it is underemphasized, the hair falls out, the nails are brittle, the teeth tend to decay, and the bones and joints are raw, weak, and painful.

Asthi Dhatu, which is formed and nourished by the *Dhatus* higher up the chain, supplies in turn *Majja Dhatu*, the bone marrow. This *Dhatu* has *Ap* (or *Jala*), water, as its basic element. When healthy, *Majja Dhatu* creates a general impression of softness and flexibility both in the physique and in the voice. Rounded, strong, and well-developed joints, activity, and a love of learning are further characteristics.

Increased *Majja Dhatu* shows itself in a feeling of heaviness and chronic ulcers around the bones. Reduced *Majja Dhatu* is seen in repeated attacks arising from increased *Vata* and in an obvious reduction in the quantity of *Sukra Dhatu*. Typical signs are pains in the bones and joints, a feeling that the bones are too light or soft, and a sensation of giddiness.

Majja Dhatu has the important task of nourishing the seventh *Dhatu*, Sukra. This *Dhatu*, simply named 'seed' in the old writings, is the reproductive material of both sexes. Its function is the transmission of life, and its basic element is *Ap* (or *Jala*), water.

A healthy condition of *Sukra* shows itself in strong sexual desires, great sensitivity, and fertility. A person whose *Sukra* is functioning well is bright, cheerful, and charming. The teeth are strong and well-formed. He or she is psychologically strong, healthy, and fundamentally happy.

An exaggerated *Sukra Dhatu* makes a man oversexed and increases his seminal flow. In women there is increased menstruation; their breasts swell and start lactating (secreting milk) spontaneously, and the nipples may feel stiff and sore. Reduced *Sukra Dhatu* shows itself in weariness and symptoms of exhausation, in a dry mouth, and in anemia. In men there is impotence; ejaculation is very brief or nonexistent and the semen may be stained with blood, the penis is tender, and the testicles ache. In women menstruation is weak and irregular and the breasts are stunted and produce little or no milk.

The seven *Dhatus* express themselves with different degrees of strength in different individuals, much as the *Tridoshas* are present in differing degrees. And just as the ruling *Dosha* will feature strongly in type-description, so the relative prominence of the *Dhatus* is important in the treatment of disease. A harmonious balance does not imply an equal division, but it does imply that the various elements are in their natural, healthy condition.

The *Tridoshas* themselves, as energy principles in the material realm, are also regarded as *Dhatus* when in balance. Thus, to the Ayurvedic physician they have the rank of an element in natural philosophy, being treated as *Doshas* (or faults) only when disharmonious or in cases of disease.

The Indians take into account the intermediate forms between material states and energy fields. Also, they see nothing strange in imagining a condition that is simultaneously a form of energy and a form of matter. The seven *Dhatus*, material though they may be, together form a true energy principle, an essence known as *Ojas Dhatu*, which has properties similar to the *Kapha* principle. Its function is plain: as the essence of all the *Dhatus*, it produces a natural radiance.

In addition to the seven *Dhatus*, to *Ojas Dhatu*, and to the *Tridoshas* (which in normal cases are taken to be *Dhatus*), we have a series of secondary *Dhatus* or *Upa Dhatus* which maintain certain organs and regions of the body. Among these are the tendons, blood vessels, nerves and nerve cells, the ligaments, skin layers, breast milk and menstrual blood, as well as the body's reserves of fat which support *Meda Dhatu* during abstention from food.

Our bodies are traversed by large and small 'channels', or transport routes requires to sustain life. Air has to be breathed in and out, food has to be ingested and digested, the nutrients need to be transported, the blood must circulate, and—to avoid poisoning the body—waste products must be excreted. The *Srotas*, the body's ducts, are the trachea, the esophagus, the stomach and intestines, and the arteries, veins, and capillaries. Even the minutest vessels belong to this group, provided they are intact and allow for continuous circulation.

Ayurveda distributes these 'channels' into thirteen different categories:

1   *Prana Vaha Srotas*: channels leading the outside air into the blood stream.

2 *Udaka Vaha Srotas*: channels transporting water, including serum and lymph.

3 *Anna Vaha Srotas*: the transport system for solid and liquid nutrients.

4 *Rasa Vaha Srotas*: the conducting system for plasma and chyle.

5 *Rakta Vaha Srotas*: channels in which hemoglobin in particular arises and circulates.

6 *Mamsa Vaha Srotas*: transport routes along which the building materials for muscle tissue are carried.

7 *Meda Vaha Srotas*: channels in which the building materials for fatty tissue are carried.

8 *Asthi Vaha Srotas*: transport routes for the building materials of bony tissue.

9 *Majja Vaha Srotas*: tributaries for the building materials of marrow.

10 *Sukra Vaha Srotas*: tributaries for the building materials of the gonads, as well as the ducts for sperm and ova.

11 *Mutra Vaha Srota*: the drainage system for urine (ureters and urethra).

12 *Purisha Vaha Srota*: the transport route for the removal of feces (colon and rectum).

13 *Sveda Vaha Srotas*: channels for perspiration (sudoriferous ducts).

For each type of channel the Ayurvedic literature specifies certain 'places of origin,' and it is at one or another of these places that symptoms of disease are observed when the circulation of a given system is disrupted. Taking them in the same order as that of their respective categories above, they are:

1 Heart, thoracic cavity, and abdominal cavity.
2 Palate, pancreas.
3 Stomach.
4 Heart, blood vessels.
5 Liver, spleen.
6 Ligaments, skin.
7 Kidneys, adipose tissue in the abdomen.
8 Bony tissue and adipose (fatty) tissue.
9 Bones and joints.
10 Testicles and ovaries.
11 Kidneys, bladder.
12 Colon, rectum.
13 Adipose tissue, hair follicles.

Certain influences affect the natural functioning of the various *Srotas*:

1 *Prana Vaha*: the suppression or uninhibited indulgence of natural needs. Physical exertions on an empty stomach. Also 'negligence in the face of bleak conditions.'

2 *Udaka Vaha*: deficient digestion, food that is too dry, great thirst, alcohol, heat.

3 *Anna Vaha*: irregular meals, indigestible food, weak digestion.

4 *Rasa Vaha*: excessive intake of heavy, cold, and greasy foodstuffs. Undue cares.

5 *Rakta Vaha*: greasy, hot foods, which stimulate and contain a considerable amount of liquid. Heat.

6 *Mamsa Vaha*: fatty coarse, and heavy food. Sleep immediately after meals.

7 *Meda Vaha*: fatty foods and lack of exercise. Sleep during the day.

8 *Asthi Vaha*: all substances that strengthen *Vata*. Physical exertions which impose too great a strain on the bones and joints.

9 *Majja Vaha*: injuries and compression of the bones. Too much liquid.

10 *Sukra Vaha*: applications of alkaline substances. Surgical operations.

11 *Mutra Vaha*: holding back the urine.

12 *Purisha Vaha*: holding back the feces. Excessive and too frequent intake of food without waiting for the last meal to be properly digested or when the digestion is weak.

13 *Sveda Vaha*: overexertion, heat, drinking too much, anger, grief, fear.

Three of these thirteen channels transport the three *Malas*, the main elimination products of the body: *Purisha* (feces), *Mutra* (urine), and *Sveda* (sweat).

In fact, there are other *Malas* arising from the various stages of metabolism, and other forms in which dead cells are discarded: the skin scales, hair falls out, and the nails break, for example. Such pieces of debris are termed *Mala Dhatus*. However, whatever their name, they are of no more than passing interest as far as we are concerned, since they do not produce disease. The three *Malas* are waste products that it is absolutely essential for the body to eliminate, and if their elimination is disturbed, the consequences can be serious.

The determining element in defecation is *Prthivi*, the earth. Any imbalance in the *Tridoshas* giving rise to an unhealthy state of the feces will reveal itself in typical symptoms. Increased *Purisha* is attended by gurgling sounds in the abdomen, by flatulence, wind, pain, and a heavy feeling. Reduced *Purisha* produces a violent agitation of *Vata*, an upward and downward movement of wind accompanied by abdominal noises, pains in the chest and around the heart, and soreness of the abdominal cavity, with throbbing pains.

The element water (*Jala* or *Ap*) and the element fire (*Tejas* or *Agni*) are the 'building blocks' of urine. Unbalanced, increased *Mutra* shows itself in a pathological increase in the amount of urine and an increased desire to pass water, together with a painful enlargement of the bladder. Reduced *Mutra* results in a reduced amount of urine. An intense thirst, dry mouth, and pains in the lower abdomen are the symptoms.

Sveda, or sweat, has water as its basic element. Increased *Sveda* shows itself in increased perspiration, itching, and an unpleasant smell. Reduced *Sveda* brings about an inability to perspire, with a tendency to dry, cracked skin, hair loss, and a lessened sensibility of the sense of touch.

13

THE BIOLOGICAL FIRE
Agni *the Fire of Life*

'*Agni* is responsible for the whole life process, for a person's appearance, for his strength, his energy, his health, for his weight increase, for *Ojas*— i.e., for his life essence and glow, for his body temperature and lifebreath.' This is how Charaka's classic text describes the comprehensive function of metabolism as conceived by Ayurveda, a concept which can be summed up in a single word: *Agni*, or fire.

As we have seen, the 'power of fire' working in the body is known as the principle *Pitta*. The question of the difference between *Pitta* and *Agni* is an interesting one. It is the difference between combustion and flame. *Pitta* is the energy of fire, whereas *Agni* is fire itself, or biological fire. When this fire is extinguished, life ends. Quite a few sayings express the old knowledge that there is a fire burning within us: '. . . the fire of life is burning high—burning low,' etc. Charaka says of *Agni*, 'Food is digested and broken down with the help of *Agni*. What we eat cannot nourish our bodies except by *Agni*. And life and death depend on *Agni's* functioning.'

One of the five forms of *Pitta*, *Pachaka Pitta* is known as the 'fire of digestion.' Can *Pachaka Pitta* be equated with *Agni* perhaps? That would be like equating a count with a king. *Pachaka Pitta* discharges its main function in the digestion of food in the stomach and intestines, whereas *Agni* controls all the metabolic processes in the body—the processes of decomposing and transforming the food, together with the processes of oxygenation and the replacement of worn tissues.

For the maintenance and improvement of health it is extremely important that *Agni* should be working properly. When its function is reduced, digestion is incomplete and metabolism is impaired. The resulting substances, consisting of imperfectly converted food, are called *Ama*, or 'unripe.' The formation of *Ama* is followed by fermentation and by putrefaction in the stomach and intestines. Most endogenous diseases—called *Amajanya*—are caused by the absorption of *Ama*. *Ama* is the sworn enemy of the *Tridoshas* and plays a significant part in upsetting their balance.

All told, there are thirteen kinds of *Agni*, of which the most important is *Jathara Agni* since this influences the functioning of all the other *Agnis*. It operates in the region of the stomach and intestines and is responsible for the digestion of food, for the absorption of nutrients, and for the formation of waste products. *Jathara Agni* is also a catalyst in the production of the digestive juices. Its role in the formation of *Ahara Rasa*, from which all the *Dhatus* arise and by which they are maintained, has been mentioned in the previous chapter.

Five more forms of *Agni* take care of the further decomposition of substances. They are known as *Bhutagni*, and their number is derived from the basic elements, the five *Mahabhutas*. Their chief site is the liver.

The seven *Dhatu Agni* are found in the tissue cells and bring about the metabolic process in this department. Their number corresponds to the number of the *Dhatus*.

A certain set of factors undermines the functioning of *Agni*. One such factor is undernourishment and another is overnourishment. Then again there is the eating of heavy or completely indigestible meals, not to mention eating to excess. Other factors are chronic diseases, emotional states like rage or grief, extremes of climate, seasonal changes, uncongenial living quarters, and whatever flys in the face of socio-cultural conventions—especially those involving dietary rules such as the abstinence from meat of the Hindus and the fasts of some sections of Christianity. Any change in eating habits is a challenge to the body, and the breaking of a taboo creates psychological stress as well. Charaka has this to say about the effects of interfering factors: 'If there are disturbances in the region of the stomach and intestines, not even the lightest food can be digested and broken down. Those substances which are not broken down turn sour and act as poisons.'

Four states of *Agni* are distinguished, according to how they behave:

- In *Mandagni*, *Kapha Dosha* predominates. The excess of *Kapha* slows digestion down and makes it weak and sluggish. *Manda* means slow and lazy and is a fundamental property of *Kapha*.
- In *Tiksnagni*, *Pitta* predominates and intensifies digestion. *Tiksna* means keen and is a fundamental property of *Pitta*.
- In *Visamagni*, *Vata* predominates and brings about great irregularity in the digestion. *Visama* means irregular and is a fundamental property of *Vata*.
- *Sama* means normal, regular, and harmonious and is a term used

to designate a well-balanced state of the *Tridoshas*. In *Samagni* there is a nicely regulated working of *Agni*.

General symptoms of defective metabolism are costiveness, dejection, headache, vertigo, debility, stiffness in the back and hips, reduced peristalsis (bowel movement), emaciation, and poor digestion. In addition, there are specific symptoms depending on the strength and localization of the disturbance. Typical diseases arising from metabolic disturbances in the region of the stomach and intestines are gastroenteritis, costiveness, chronic gastritis, and colitis.

Amavata is one of the diseases mentioned in the *Madhava Nidana*, an important medical treatise of the seventh century. We know it today as synovitis, that is to say, an inflammation of the synovial membrane, a form of arthritis. Here *Ama* works on *Kapha* first of all, but it is the symptoms of pain that have put the word *Vata* into the name of the disease, which has much in common with *Vatarakta*, a disorder with the same symptoms as gout. Another group of diseases goes under the name *Samtaprana*; among them are obesity and diabetes mellitus. *Bhasmaka* is a form of disease in which the symptoms are like those of hyperthyrosis (excessive secretion from the thyroid gland) or thyrotoxicosis (poisoning from excessive secretion of the thyroid gland) as the case may be.

Therapy includes herbs, diet, and physical and mental exercises. It concentrates mainly on the region of the stomach and intestines and on the most important *Agni* operative there—*Jathara Agni*.

The detoxifying, cleansing diet might consist, for example, of a wheat breakfast cereal plus medicinal herbs to improve the digestion and accelerate excretion. Examples of such herbs are herbal bitters or fennel, caraway, aniseed, and ginger.

The struggle against the 'death fiend' *Ama* also figures in European folk lore, as anyone can see who cares to leaf back through our centuries-old literature. 'Death dwells in the bowels,' was a household saying in ancient Europe.

14

WE ARE WHAT WE EAT
The Importance of Diet

The great vibrating harmony that links the macrocosm with each individual living microcosm was our starting point in describing the Ayurvedic view of humanity. Yet, it is not only man who is a microcosm: each plant, too, is a tiny reflection of that macrocosm we call the universe, and contains all the elements that go to make up the mighty cosmos. And active in each plant are the three energy principles found at work in all other living things.

The chief significance of plants for human beings is their function as food; and, of course; they are significant in exactly the same way for every animal, whether carniverous or not, since plants are invariably found at the beginning of the food chain. Nevertheless, in the widest sense of the term, everything we take from our environment is nourishment. The different qualities of what we 'feed on' have quite specific effects on us.

Each individual is born with a predetermined basic pattern of the building blocks of being. His *Tridoshas* and his character type are all part of this pattern. However, the balance is finely poised, and changes big and small cause it to swing this way and that all through life.

However, not only are we constantly assimilating the world; we are constantly shedding our life-energy with every act and movement. As our cells die new ones replace them. Nothing is ever at a standstill, and all the transformations taking place in our bodies are controlled by *Agni*, the biological Fire. Metaphorically speaking, *Agni* 'devours' the fundamental elements. This natural loss has to be made good in order to preserve the delicate balance of the system. We recoup it by food and drink, by gratification of the senses, by light and fresh air, and by spiritual activity.

As far as Ayurveda is concerned, this means that any disharmony in the body can be treated by what we eat. Foods are remedies, plants are healing drugs, and diet is the best therapy. Now, to our ears, the word 'diet' may not sound particularly inviting. It has an ominously unpleasant ring about it, and conjures up visions of lean rations and uninteresting fare. However, that is the negative European tradition. The phrase 'bitter medicine' goes back to the Middle Ages when illnesses were thought to be meted out by Divine justice and sweet things would have seemed singularly inappropriate as remedies. It was argued that, if the remedy tasted nasty enough to become part of the punishment, God would accordingly shorten the time of suffering under the disease. A palatable preparation would not have been credited with healing power, and a doctor who did not carry a bag full of medical instruments of torture would have inspired little confidence. In principle, this attitude hasn't changed. A certain masochism is encountered in modern patients, too.

The dieting craze in industrialized countries is really all part of the same pattern. We have weight loss and detoxification diets and macrobiotic and dietetic advice handed out by Brucker, Schnitzer, Atkins, or Hay—all of it contradictory. However, the various regimes do have this in common—the intake of food is very closely monitored, and patients suffer a measure of deprivation which can eventually result in deficiency symptoms and may even prove dangerous.

However, I should like to take a closer look at one dietary theory because of its interesting similarity to what we find in Ayurveda. I am speaking of *Sattvik* theory as expounded by the Buddhists and, since Buddhism originated in northern India, the similarity is not accidental. *Sattvik* theory divides foodstuffs into three categories: *Sattvik*, *Rajsik*, or *Tamsik*. We have already met the stems of these three words in *Sattwa*, *Rajas*, and *Tamas*, the three basic elements of *Prakrti* (nature, or the matter principle) and then in a further manifestation as the three qualities of *Manas* (the human mind), which determine the way in which the mind expresses itself.

Sattwa means balance, spiritual life, and right dealing—the very things for which Buddhism strives. *Rajas* means energy which, although essential, can work positively in the direction of *Sattwa* or negatively in the direction of *Tamas*. *Tamas* itself means inertia, dullness, and heaviness (of body or mind).

Sattvik nourishment includes all vegetable foodstuffs (except spices) and cow's milk. According to *Sattvik* teaching, these should form the staple articles of diet. *Rajsik* nourishment consists of permissible energy-giving foods, including animal milk products, to prevent deficiency diseases and energy loss. *Tamsik* nourishment is the meat of dead animals, rejected by many Buddhists because of the prohibition against taking life.

Sattvik theory is no narrow sectarian doctrine but presents us with guidelines for sensible eating. It does not advocate severe fasts but regards eating as a positive, joyful, intelligent activity. Fasting, if it is done at all, is something voluntary that is undertaken at special stages of spiritual development.

Turning now to what Ayurveda has to say about eating, we cannot fail to be struck by the surprising fact that Hindu eating habits vary considerably from the proposals found in Ayurveda. In Hinduism (as in its offshoot, Buddhism), meat is refused as a form of nourishment. Strict Hindus do not eat fish or even eggs. Nevertheless, allowances have always been made for environmental conditions. Thus, Hindus living by the sea are allowed to eat fish three times a week. Or, to look at another modification, the Brahmins of Bengal count fish as plant food. And throughout India the rule is that the lower the caste—or, which comes to much the same thing, the poorer the person—the less stringent are the dietary laws and taboos. This is obviously a matter of necessity; it is relatively easy for wealthy Brahmins to secure a well-balanced diet of vegetables and fruit, supplemented by nutritious clarified butter (ghee) and plenty of milk.

Ayurveda, the doctrine of how to live life to the full, is not bound by religious rules and regulations but concerns itself with the requirements of the human body and the latter's need of the correct amounts of proteins, carbohydrates, fats, vitamins, minerals, and so on. In the Ayurvedic texts there are descriptions of the effects of all kinds of meats on the *Tridoshas*.

Generally speaking, Ayurveda stresses the value of a well-chosen, balanced diet containing all six tastes. An excess of one or another of the tastes—in a prescribed diet—is introduced on occasion to meet the special needs of a healthy or ill individual, of an expectant mother or a child, of someone doing heavy manual work, or of the person in a sedentary occupation. The relationship of the tastes to the three bioenergetic principles has already been described; here we are more interested in their bearing on diet because it is very useful to us to be able to assess what we are eating from its flavor.

Ayurveda underlines the importance of taking freshly prepared hot meals because they are easily digested, stimulate the flow of digestive juices, and encourage a steady rate of peristalsis. There are also other Ayurvedic recommendations for keeping disease at bay:

- No more should be eaten until the last meal has been completely digested.

- The type of food should suit the time of year. For instance, during the cold season, more sweet and sour foods should be consumed, i.e., more carbohydrates, fats or oils, and vitamin-rich items.
- The amount eaten must just satisfy and depends on the individual digestive power of *Agni*.
- Meals should not be eaten too quickly or too slowly. The act of eating should engage the eater's undivided attention.
- The circumstances in which meals are taken are important too— the place, the people, the atmosphere of the place. Congenial surroundings are very salutary.

Foodstuffs are divided into twelve groups: cereals, legumes, flesh, vegetables growing under the ground, fruit, nuts, wine, water, milk, sugar, fats and oils, and spices. Prepared dishes are placed in four categories:

1 Foods of normal consistency, such as rice or bread.
2 Liquid foods, such as vegetable or meat soup, fruit juice, milk, etc.
3 Tasty foods, such as ketchups and pastes, preserves, chutneys, and sweet and sour sauce, designed to tickle the palate.
4 Crisp and chewy foods, such as salads or nuts.

To give the body what it needs, our daily diet should include foods from all four of the above groups. Above all, we ought to keep a careful eye on the quality of what we are eating. White flour, husked and polished rice, white sugar, and chemically treated fruit and meat should be avoided.

As we see then, Ayurvedic dietary theory can hardly be called narrow. The kind of diet it proposes is not restrictive but enriches life. It is a diet adapted to the individual's makeup, to the energy conditions basic to his nature, to the expression of the *Tridoshas*; it has an equalizing effect and takes into account not only the state of health but the time of day, the time of year, and the dieter's age. It maximizes energy and does not draw on the body's reserves. By using the correct diet, the body can be used to full capacity without hurting the joints, tendons, and muscles. The working of the mind is enhanced, too. Because of the flexibility and high-energy potential of the diet, the individual is left untrammeled. There is no need to be abstemious or to make do with food substitutes. A diet of this sort can only increase enjoyment and prolong life.

15

WHAT DOES THE UNIVERSE TASTE LIKE?
An Alternative Mode of Knowing

Dravyaguna is the name given to the identification, classification, and knowledge of the properties of foods, remedies, drugs, and diets. The word *Dravya* means 'substance', 'stuff', 'matter'; the word *Guna* means 'quality', as we have already seen.

In order to obtain an understanding of this complex system, we must know a few more Sanskrit words from the *Nyaya Vaisesika*. These are: *Karma*, or 'effect', 'movement', *Samanya*, or 'sameness'; *Visesa*, or 'antagonism', 'diversity'; and *Samavaya*, 'inseparable inherence.'

A medicinal plant, *Dravya* is characterized by its qualities (*Gunas*) and by the effects (*Karma*) of these. Quality and effect cannot exist apart from substance, in which they inhere inseparably (*Samavaya*). A drug may act on the homeopathic principle of sameness (*Samanya*) or on the allopathic principle of antagonism (*Visesa*). In Ayurvedic practice, for example, substances with the property 'hot' have a heating effect and accelerate metabolism; they strengthen *Pitta* by the principle of sameness and reduce *Kapha* by the principle of antagonism.

But the building blocks of existence, the *Mahabhutas*, are operative, too. For instance, substances in which the elements earth and water predominate are assimilated by body tissues composed of the same elements. Substance and tissue fit each other, in this case, like lock and key.

Many of the Indian methods of classifying remedies are similar to our own:

1   Classification according to mode of application, either as diet (high dosage) or as medication (low dosage).
2   Classification according to the origin of the animal, vegetable, and mineral preparations concerned, with all that this entails from a scientific point of view.
3   Classification according to therapeutic use relative to the *Tridoshas*. This classification is found only in Ayurveda, there being nothing

comparable in other systems of medicine. Medications function either as *Samsamana*, symptomatically, that is to say they calm the Doshas, or as *Samsodhana*, in which case they clean an excess of Doshas out of the body. In so-called *Panchakarma* therapy,[29] the *Samsodhana* action is obtained by five possible methods of elimination: *Vamana* (vomiting), *Virecana* (purging), *Anuvasana* (oily enemas), *Niruhana* (dry enemas), and *Sirovirecana* (errhines). Detailed classifications of medicaments employed in *Panchakarma* therapy are to be found in the ancient texts.

4 Classification according to pharmacological action. Charaka enumerates fifty groups of ten plants each.
5 Classification according to pharmacological action and therapeutic use. Susruta mentions thirty-seven groups.

European medicine has something corresponding to each of these methods of classification—with the exception of number three—but Ayurveda's most important method of classification is unique: the classification of remedies according to their elemental composition. And this classification on the basis of the 'elements' is made entirely through the sense of taste.

Each taste is composed of two fundamental elements, so before we examine the effects of the six tastes we must be clear about the effects of each of the elements which, though themselves without any obvious flavor, determine the various flavors.

As we already know, all five elements invariably occur together, although not in equal proportions because one or another of them predominates at a given time. Therefore, medicinal plants can be divided into five groups with typical properties and effects. The sense of taste is the instrument used to discriminate between them, and *Rasa* or 'taste', indicates how the elements combine.

We have already encountered the Sanskrit word *Rasa* as a name for one of the seven body tissues, the *Dhatus*. The ambiguity of the Sanskrit terms is explained as follows by Dr. R. Lobo, using *Rasa* (which means both 'lymph' and 'taste') as an example: 'The Indian word for the life-supporting fluid of the internal and external environment is *Rasa*. It means not only the lymph which bathes the cells of our bodies, but also the food-essence detected by our sense of taste and instinctively sought by our appetites to maintain the total environment within our bodies. Appetite in this sense of the word is the point of intersection of constitution, education, weather change, seasonal variation, and of the body's internal economy, of the endogenous rhythms— and is thus a very complex regulator of our behaviour and not simply of the process of eating. What is more, there are an intellectual appetite and an emotional appetite, which are just as important to satisfy as are our purely physical food requirements.'[30]

Characteristics of Substances, Classified According to the Fundamental Elements[31]

Group	Taste (Rasa)	Properties (Guna)	Effects (Karma)
earthy (*parthiva*)	sweet (and slightly astringent)	heavy, rough, hard, inert, stable, clear, dense, coarse	promotes growth, weight, compactness, stability, strength—downward movements: aperient
water (*apya*)	sweet (and slightly astringent, sour, and salty)	cold, oily, inert, mobile, fluid, soft, gelatinous	moistening, lubricating, binding, solvent, pleasantly cooling
fiery (*taijasa*)	pungent (and slightly sour and salty)	hot, pungent, fine, dry, rough, light, clear	burning, digestive, energy-giving, heating, radiant, purifying—upward movement: emetic
airy (*vayavya*)	astringent (and slightly bitter)	fine, rough, cold, light, clear	purifying, drying, loosening, alleviating, tiring, promoting movement
etheric (*akasiya*)	unmanifest	smooth, subtle, soft, clear, light, separating	softening, unblocking (duct cleaning)

Several indications are immediately apparent from the above fundamental list. To promote growth and weight increase, an 'earthy' drug is given, and a 'watery' one is given when there has been a considerable loss of body fluid. A 'fiery' drug stimulates the digestive fire *Agni* when the stomach is disordered. An 'airy' drug can aid dieting, and 'etheric' drugs open and cleanse the channels, or the *Srotas*.

As far as therapy is concerned, the most important properties of the elements are as follows: in earth, 'weight'; in water 'lubrication'; in fire, 'stimulation'; in air 'roughness'; and in ether, 'lightness'.

Taste perception of how the elements combine in various substances is unparalleled and unique* and is known only to the Ayurvedic system. Taking the sense of taste as a starting point, a comprehensive system has been developed that classifies plants according to their effects, with further reference to the changes undergone by plant constituents in the body and to the alterations in action produced by these changes.

In highly industrialized regions, problems are certainly encountered with a scientific system that does not trust the human senses. 'Whereas we make no bones about accepting the subjective taste of a person where fashion, individual life-style and the quality of human relationships are concerned, the attempt to use taste as a standard of classification would be branded as unscientific.'[32] The grotesque attitude so described has been adopted to the extent that we have almost ceased to trust our natural faculties of perception: they have been dulled by our reliance on so-called 'superior' technology and mechanically oriented knowledge. A regression of the senses is in full swing.

Now the sense of taste, which is the most important instrument possessed by Ayurveda for perceiving the healing quality of a substance, has become badly distorted in Western society. The almost tasteless banana and battery-reared fowls dominate the market. There is much the same levelling in what we put in our stomachs as there is in architecture. The tasteless painkiller is a good symbol of the deadening of all direct contact with reality through the sense organs.

The American psychotherapists Erving and Miriam Polster were made very much aware of this predicament in their practice and remarked: 'We have reached the point where taste has been sacrificed for the sake of convenience and profit. Fewer and fewer people are aware of the

---

* Translator's note: Ancient Greek and Roman physicians, however, classified herbal remedies according to taste and also according to whether they were 'hot', 'dry', 'moist' to various degrees. An acrid taste, for example, was counted as hot, whereas an acid taste was not. Culpeper, in his 'herbal', still adheres to this old system in part.

great gulf dividing mass-produced from home-made food. And even when they are aware of it, they have no time to trouble themselves over it or else they feel the matter is too trivial.' And, in another passage, they come to the following conclusion: 'Foregoing the simple, fundamental contact opportunities offered us in the taste of food is only a short step away from devaluing contact in general.'[33]

Yet what is so extraordinary is that if we want to lodge an appeal for more reliance to be placed in the sense of taste, Western science itself can be called to the witness stand as evidence for the propriety of the Ayurvedic position. Even though technological civilization may have blunted our five senses, the very principle of accurate product control has brought highly qualified specialists to the fore—well-paid food tasters whose delicate palates can precisely detect the sulphite content in treated raisins, the water percentage in raw marzipan, or the amount of lead in canned foods. International scientists have given their blessings to this method of testing, since its results are usually more reliable than those of chemical analysis. 'Experience teaches that a result is more trustworthy the more straightforwardly it is obtained.'[34]

Even if we are not food tasters, we do have our own taste preferences which guide us in the choice of food which is right for us. Provided we do not have a perverted appetite for unwholesome food, we shall find that there is little enjoyment in fruit with a reduced vitamin C content, and that when fruit and vegetables are much contaminated with pesticides they lose their typical flavors. These are facts that ought to bolster our confidence in our sense of taste and encourage us to use it as a regulator of communication in the on-going dialogue between man and his environment, between microcosm and macrocosm.

The entire universe is constructed from the building blocks of being. Whoever knows how these building blocks, or elements, taste knows how the universe tastes. No machine will ever discover it for us. In order to be able to differentiate between the various ways in which remedies act from the time they are taken to their final effect, we shall need to use some further concepts. While *Rasa* is the basic taste of a substance, *Vipaka* is that taste after it has been changed by digestion and transformation in the body. While *Guna* is the physical property of a substance, *Virya* is the potency that evokes a reaction in the body; in other words, it is the drug action. *Prabhava* is a mysterious specific effect which is not logically derivable from *Rasa*. And *Anurasa* is the name for any fugitive flavor in fresh fruit or vegetables that produces no obvious reaction.

The recognized tastes are six in number, each being formed from some two of the elements:

TASTE		ELEMENT	
sweet	(*madhura*)	earth, water	(*Prthivi, Jala*)
sour	(*amla*)	earth, fire	(*Prthivi, Tejas*)
salty	(*lavana*)	water, fire	(*Jala, Tejas*)
pungent	(*katu*)	air, fire	(*Vayu, Tejas*)
bitter	(*tikta*)	air, ether	(*Vayu, Akasha*)
astringent	(*kasaya*)	air, earth	(*Vayu, Prthivi*)

Roughly speaking, the chemical correspondences are as follows:

TASTE	SUBSTANCES
sweet	*carbohydrates, sugars, fats, amino acids*
sour	*organic acids*
salty	*salts*
pungent	*volatile oils*
bitter	*bitter principles, alkaloids, glycosides*
astringent	*tannin*

The way in which the six tastes are made up of the elements has been worked out empirically from observations of their action on the body. For example, 'sweet' (*madhura*), with its leading elements earth and water, is a builder of those tissues that are formed from earth and water. A sweet-tasting substance will strengthen *Kapha Dosha*, which is itself composed of earth and water, but will weaken *Pitta Dosha* (made from the element fire) and *Vata Dosha* (made from air and ether).

The effects of medications on the *Tridoshas* can therefore be discovered from their tastes:

TASTE weakening the *Dosha*	DOSHA	TASTE strengthening the *Dosha*
sweet		pungent
sour	*VATA*	bitter
salty		astringent
sweet		sour
bitter	*PITTA*	salt
astringent		pungent
pungent		sweet
bitter	*KAPHA*	sour
astringent		salty

The final outcome depends on the interaction of the elements in the six tastes with those in the three *Doshas*.

The three tastes containing the element fire (sour, salty, and pungent) strengthen *Pitta*; that is to say, they strengthen all those functions associated with a rise in temperature, all metabolic processes such as the digestion of food, pigmentation of the blood, and the formation of various secretions and excretions as the end products of tissue combustion. The tastes that do not contain the element fire weaken *Pitta*.

The three tastes containing the element air (pungent, bitter, astringent) strengthen and increase *Vata* and all phenomena to do with movement, penetration, and cleansing of the channels. On the other hand, the tastes that do not contain the element air (sweet, sour, salty) weaken *Vata* and sedate it but strengthen *Kapha*.

A strengthening action is exercised on *Kapha* by the tastes sweet, sour, and salty because they contain one or both of the elements earth and water (like *Kapha* itself). The tastes pungent, bitter, and astringent sedate *Kapha*, weaken it, and normalize it. It is true that the element

Classification of Medications
by the Six Tastes,
Their Qualities, and Effects [35]

Taste	Quality	EFFECTS		
		on the three forces	positive	negative
sweet	oily, cold, heavy	K P, V	promotes weight increase, vitalizes, has an aperient and diuretic action	obesity, respiratory disorders, anorexia, goiter, swelling of the lymph nodes, worms, diabetes
sour	oily, hot, heavy	K, P V	stimulates the appetite, promotes digestion, expels wind, combats anorexia	blood disorders, swellings, inflammations, flushing, anemia, hemmorhage, nausea, visual disorders

salty	oily, hot, heavy	K, P V	moistens, stimulates the appetite promotes digestion, expectorant, breaks up	impotence, greying and falling hair, bleeding, stomach disorders skin diseases
pungent	rough, hot, light	V, P K	stimulates the appetite, cleans the mouth, promotes digestion, promotes weight loss, vermifuge	impotence, unconsciousness, nausea, mental weekness, hot feeling, thirst
bitter	rough, cold, light	V P, K	stimulates the appetite, promotes digestion, vermifuge, febrifuge, antitoxic	consumption, mental weakness, nausea, dry mouth, nervous disorders
astringent	rough, cold, light	V P, K	astringes, absorbs, anti-inflammatory	heart trouble, dry mouth, clogging through contraction of the canals, impotence, nerve disorders

earth enters into the composition of the taste astringent, but air is its leading element, as it is of the tastes pungent and bitter. What strengthens Vata weakens *Kapha* and vice versa.

The *Rasas* have an immediate effect. Reactions are observable as soon as the remedies are taken; there is a feeling of satisfaction or well-being. However, this effect is localized and lasts no longer than the time needed to initiate biochemical changes in the body. The process of digesting a substance often breaks the dominance of the leading element, and a new tendency known as *Vipaka* appears.

This secondary action is delayed and is not local but is systemic, that is to say, it affects the whole body. The mental responses take some time to show themselves, too. *Rasa* and *Vipaka* represent two successive stages in the action of a medication. As soon as the first stage ends, the second begins. Therefore, a knowledge of how *Vipaka* works is essential for anyone engaging in therapy.

The classical authors Susruta and Charaka describe the action of *Vipaka* from different points of view, but their findings are in full agreement with one another. Susruta distinguishes two main groups of *Vipaka* based on the contrasting properties heavy and light. Heavy *Vipaka* has an anabolic effect and builds up the tissues. Light *Vipaka* is catabolic and breaks down the body's tissues. Charaka, for his part, divides *Vipaka* into three groups according to the three Doshas:

Taste		Action on	
	Tridoshas	Tissues	Digestion
sweet	strengthens *Kapha*	builds up	—
sour	strengthens *Pitta*	breaks down	aperient
pungent	strengthens *Vata*		constipating

Sour and pungent are distinguished in *Vipaka* by their action on the digestion. In *Vipaka* the original six tastes are reduced to three: sweet and salt become sweet *Vipaka*, pungent, bitter, and astringent give rise to pungent *Vipaka*, and sour remains sour.

The *Gunas* of the ingested substances have an extremely important part to play in this change. Remedies with the property 'oily' exhibit the same action as those with a *Vipaka* which is sweet; that is to say, they are anabolic. Substances that are 'rough' exhibit the same action as those with a pungent *Vipaka*; that is to say, they are catabolic.

Guna, the physical and pharmacological property of a plant or substance, is just as important as *Rasa*, or taste, in making an accurate choice of medication. The taste tells us about the tendency of the therapeutic action; the *Guna* decides the potential action and produces inside the body qualities similar to those possessed by itself outside the body. Therefore, to take an example, or plant or mineral with the physical property heavy (*guru*) would be prescribed to increase body weight since heaviness is a property of weight.

The basic properties (or qualities) are expressed as adjectives because they are an integral part of the substance and of its potential action. A set of no more than ten contrasting pairs covers the entire range of medical action.

The Ten Contrasting Pairs of Gunas

1	*guru*	heavy	*laghu*	light
2	*sita*	cold	*ushna*	hot
3	*snigdha*	oily, viscous	*ruksa*	dry, rough, abrasive
4	*manda*	mild, slow, inactive	*tiksna*	keen, quick active
5	*sthira*	compact, static	*sara*	mobile, fluent
6	*kathina*	hard	*mrdu*	soft
7	*picchila*	slimy, gelatinous, sticky, turbid	*visada*	clear, transparent
8	*slaksna*	smooth	*khara*	rough
9	*sthula*	gross, bulky	*suksma*	minute, fine, penetrating
10	*sandra*	solid, compact, dense	*drava*	liquid

These qualities are, in fact, more significant than tastes. To illustrate this point, take a glass of water. The natural taste of fresh water is 'sweet', and it accordingly stimulates and strengthens *Kapha*. But if we heat the water, it will pacify and reduce *Kapha*. The water is still sweet, but now the added property 'hot' (*ushna*) dominates.

In certain materials the basic quality enhances the action of the taste considerably. A stock example is the plant *Amalaki* (*Emblica officinalis*). As we may gather from its Sanskrit name, it has a sour taste (*amla*). Now the medicinal action indicated by this particular taste is much intensified by the properties cold and soft.

What is more, *Vipaka*, the taste as changed by digestion, frequently depends on the mode of action of the *Gunas*. Thus, substances with the properties heavy, cold, oily, and slimy become heavy in the *Vipaka* form, but substances which are light, hot, rough, and clear are light in the *Vipaka* form.

Finally, the sheer variety of applications indicated by the *Gunas* gives them a decided advantage over the simple division into tastes since the *Gunas* are a guide to external as well as internal use, whereas the tastes are a guide to internal use only.

For instance, the heating action of the property 'hot' can regulate the digestion by strengthening *Agni*, and in the form of hot compresses can relieve cramps and can draw the matter out of boils. Or, again, the property 'oily' is laxative or lubricating internally, and is useful in massage externally.

The following tables provides a general synopsis of the twenty properties or qualities (*Gunas*), of their component elements (*Mahabhutas*), of their effect on the *Tridoshas*, and of the tendency of their main action.

Property	Elements	Action on the *Tridoshas* ↑	Action on the *Tridoshas* ↓	Tendency of the Principal Effect
1 heavy	earth, water	K	V	weight increasing
2 light	fire, air, ether	V	K	weight reducing
3 cold	water	V, K	P	cooling
4 hot	fire	P	V, K	heating
5 oily	water	K	V	moistening
6 dry	earth, fire, air	V	K	absorptive
7 mild	earth, water	K	P	retarding
8 keen	fire	P	K	intensifying accelerating
9 compact	earth	K		stabilizing
10 mobile	air	K		moving, mobilizing
11 soft	water, ether	K		emollient (softening)
12 hard	earth	V		indurative (hardening)
13 clean	earth, fire, air, ether	V		cleansing
14 slimy	water	K		lubricating, oiling
15 smooth	fire	P		soothing, healing
16 rough	air	V		roughening
17 minute	fire, air, ether	V		penetrating
18 gross	earth	K		clogging
19 solid	earth	K		solidifying
20 liquid	water	K		liquefying

The following synopsis gives examples of remedies exhibiting the principal effects of the *Gunas*. The plants mentioned all grow, or are obtainable, in Europe.

1	weight increasing	Essential foodstuffs such as corn, potatoes, or legumes.
2	weight reducing	Drugs promoting digestion: plants containing essential oils; seaweed. Agents that detoxify by regulating bowel action: wheat bran. Diuretics: juniper berries, leaves containing tannin and having an astringent taste.
3	cooling	Menthol, eucalyptus, sandalwood oil, daisy, houseleek, vine shoots.
4	heating	Diaphoretics: elderflower tea, limeflower tea. Agents that warm the stomach: essential oils such as Venetian oil of turpentine. Warming seeds: fennel, anise, caraway. External application: mustard plasters.
5	moistening	In dry coughs: liquorice (liquorice sticks and cough sweets). To liquefy and loosen the phlegm in bronchitis: plants containing saponin and mucilage, i.e., soapwort, primrose, violet. Expectorants: coltsfoot, onion, and lungwort.
6	absorptive	Powdered rice or wheat starch, lycopodium powder (spores), powdered sage leaves, fenugreek. In intestinal infections: charcoal or wheat or rice gruel.
7	retarding	Yoghurt. Tranquilizing: hops, valerian, camomile, honey.
8	intensifying (accelerating)	Rosemary. Stimulating: daisy, vine shoots, wormwood, hyssop. Reviving: sea buckthorn, wood sorrel, oats. Stimulating the circulation of the blood: sweet calamus, garlic, mistletoe, common yarrow, juniper. Promoting metabolism: stinging nettle, watercress, mistletoe, wood sorrel, wormwood, tarragon.

9	stabilizing	Banana, apple. To treat diarrhoea: oak bark, bloodwort (tormentil). To stabilize mind as well as body: marigold, dead nettle.
10	moving	For the motions: laxatives such as black alder bark, rhubarb root, aloes, senna leaves, etc.
11	emollient (softening)	Linseed oil, various fats. Mucilaginous drugs: marshmallow and other mallows.
12	indurative (hardening)	Lime for bones and teeth. Comfrey, oats, millet, horsetail.
13	cleansing	Alum. Wound-cleaning: marigold, arnica. Blood purifying: juniper berries, soapwort.
14	lubricating	Linseed oil, mucilaginous drugs, gelatine, gum arabic.
15	healing (accelerating)	Vulnerary (woundhealing): arnica, lady's mantle.
16	roughening, counter-irritant	Mustard plaster (irritating the skin).
17	penetrating	Alcohol, grape sugar (dextrose), essential oils.
18	clogging	'Superfine' flour, white sugar (puddings and pastries).
19	solidifying	Butter, fats.
20	liquefying	Milk, water.

Each property or basic quality also has a potential effect, but it is not every potential effect that reaches manifestation. The active power of a medication is known as *Virya*. The property (*Guna*) of a substance becomes curative (*Virya*) as soon as it is activated.

The classification of medications by their properties or qualities is a classification according to their potential energies and not according to the effects they actually produce (the *Virya*). However, the latter are what is really important. A substance may have a number of apparently useful qualities, but to be curative it must be capable of displaying *Virya*.

Whether or not a plant with healing potential also possesses *Virya* depends on the most varied factors. Thus, the nature of the soil in

which the plant is growing is very important. For example, plants with
an aperient action are gathered from soils of which the basic elements
are earth and water. On the other hand, plants with an emetic action
are best when gathered from soils in which the elements fire and ether
prevail.

The fact that the potency of medicinal plants depends, among other
things, on soil structure and on the state of the land where they are
growing is a truth that should be heeded in a period when the ground
is still being used as a dump for chemical fertilizers regardless of the
erosion they cause. In the classical texts of Charaka and Susruta an
ideal site for medicinal plants is described: 'Land of this type should
be level, free from large holes, stones and ant-hills, and should be well
away from the places of burning, from temples and from much
frequented localities. Its soil should flow easily, and be soft yet firm;
it ought to be black, brown, or red, have grass growing on it, be
unploughed and not occupied by large trees. And it should be well
watered.'

Another point taken up by the classical texts is the exact time of
year for picking certain plant materials. Plants which are *sita Virya*,
with a *Guna sita* manifesting itself as cold and cooling, have to be
gathered in the cold season,[36] at a time when the earth is losing energy.
On the other hand, plants which are *ushna Virya*, with a *Guna ushna*
manifesting itself as hot, are gathered in the hot season,[37] at a time
when the earth is gaining energy.

The classics also mention the ideal condition of a medicinal plant.
It ought to be fresh and not damaged by insects, poison, a harsh
environment, or inclement weather. It should be free from dirt, have
a well-developed root or rootsystem, be fully mature, and possess its
characteristic taste, color, and smell. Also, it should have been grown
during the time of year most favorable for it.

Proper storage is important to preserve the strength of medicinal
substances. For this purpose the classical texts recommend cloth bags
or earthenware pots set on wooden stands in clean, well-aired (but not
draughty) rooms with doors facing north and east.

The storage time is crucial. Raw drugs, apart from one or two
exceptions such as honey, should always be used fresh. Powdered
materials remain effective for approximately two months, ointments
for four months, and rolled pills for up to a year. On the other hand,
alcoholic and metallic preparations increase in potency as they age.

All the above factors are significant, and their nonobservance,
incorrect harvesting, and storage, or faulty preparation, lead to loss of

Virya. It must also be remembered that sometimes the active principle is confined to certain parts of the plant, and sometimes various parts contain different active principles having different effects. And, once again, we must stress that a medication can lose its virtue after a certain period of time.

There are various ways of schematizing remedies according to their medicinal action. A much-employed method is based on a set of eight basic properties. These are those properties which invariably exert an action and are always curative (*Virya*): heavy, light, cold, hot, oily, dry, soft, keen. Thus, four of the ten contrasting pairs of properties have a medicinal action in every case, and a plant with one of these properties can also exert the influence of its other *Gunas*.

Another method of classification by medicinal action is that based on the six forms of therapy:

1 *Guru virya* (heavy) helps the patient to put on weight in *Brimhana* therapy and promotes nutrition as a curative measure.
2 *Laghu virya* (light) breaks down the tissues and removes body waste in *Langhana* therapy, which heals by helping the patient to lose weight.
3 *Sita virya* (cold) is cooling and is employed in *Sthambana* therapy.
4 *Usna virya* (hot) is heating and is employed in *Svedana* sudation (sweating) therapy.
5 *Snigdha virya* (oily) is used in *Snehana* oil therapy.
6 *Ruksa virya* (dry) has a drying effect in *Ruksana* therapy.

For everyday use a division in terms of the two most popular healing properties, hot and cold, will suffice. On the plane of the *Tridoshas*, the heating effect represents *Pitta*, and the cooling effect represents *Kapha*, while *Vata* acts as a catalyst when necessary.

Substances with a sweet flavor which remain sweet after digestion (*Vipaka*) generally have a cooling effect. Substances with a sour or bitter flavor and *Vipaka* have a heating effect.

Nevertheless, as we have come to expect with rules, there are certain exceptions. For instance, the very potent plant *Amalaki* (*Emblica officinalis*) has a medicinal action which is definitely not heating even though its taste is sour before and after digestion. Flesh foods are another exception. Their basic taste is sweet and remains sweet after digestion, which would lead one to suppose that they have a cooling effect, and yet they are heating.

Internally, the heating property stimulates digestion, metabolism, and blood circulation. Externally, it can be applied for muscular and nerve pains.

The cooling property, used internally, slows down digestion, metabolism, and blood circulation. It is applied externally in fevers, swellings, and sprains (possibly accompanied by massage).

It can happen that two medicinal plants, which are completely the same in their taste both before and after digestion and are the same in their healing energies, will have differing (and sometimes quite opposite) therapeutic effects. When the therapeutic effect of a plant is different from what would be inferred from all the rules, the explanation is found in *Prabhava*. *Prabhava* means that the plant does not work in a general fashion on the *Tridoshas*, but works instead on a given tissue or organ or against a particular disease. Apparently, this *Prabhava* is what we would term the pharmacological action of a substance.

Whereas the taste, the potential property, the healing property, and the taste after digestion act directly on the bioenergetic principles, the tissues, and the excretions, and thus on the causes of disease as well as on the body and mind as a whole—in other words, they affect the entire lifesystem of an individual—*Prabhava* acts only on a specific organ or symptom. Among those remedies that work through *Prabhava* we may include emetics, laxatives, cardiac stimulants, vermifuges, and narcotics.

Without wishing to play down the value of *Prabhava* treatment, especially in specific cases, we are compelled to point out that it has its limitations. It cannot be denied that this is the aspect of Indian medicine that comes closest to the practice in modern industrialized societies. In the West, the pharmacological action of drugs on organs and cells or on pathogenic agents is given pride of place in therapy, but in Ayurvedic medicine the *Prabhava* effect is regarded as a limited option subsidiary to the main lines of treatment.

As far as the total action (or *karma*) of a medication is concerned, the general rule is that *Rasa*, the taste, gives way to *Vipaka*, the taste after digestion, just as *Vipaka* gives way to *Virya*, the potency, and *Virya* to *Prabhava*, the pharmacological action. *Karma* itself is the result of all these taken together.

16

PARALLELS IN THE WEST
Galen's Pharmacology

In the days before technology came into its own, European medicine itself was dependent on direct perception through the senses. Empirical knowledge and sensory perception were the only means by which physicians could evaluate medicinal plants for professional purposes. When the Graeco-Roman doctor, Galen (AD 129-199), personal physician to the emperor Marcus Aurelius, first worked out a comprehensive systematization of medicinal plants, he took the writings of the ancient Greeks and Romans as his authorities.[38]

I have already pointed out that a continuous exchange took place between the cultural centers of the ancient world in the form of a subtle interpenetration. Therefore, when Galen gathered together the centuries-old knowledge of his own part of the world, it is not surprising that in its main outlines his work should display definite parallels to Ayurvedic knowledge.

Galen took as his starting point the four elements of Empedocles— earth, water, fire, and air—with their qualities of dry, moist, hot, and cold. The universe is constructed out of these four elements and is stamped with their qualities. From this realization there developed the humoral pathology of the ancient Greek medical experts. The following diagram shows the relationships between the four elements, the four qualities, the cardinal humors with their organs, and the associated temperaments.

Consequently, a medicinal plant made of the four elements is able to influence the balance of the four humors when one of its basic qualities is more pronounced than the others. Now Galen innovated by going beyond a mere empirical knowledge of characteristics in order to classify plants systematically according to these basic qualities and to determine their action on the body. By taking as guidelines the doctrine of the four elements and the primary qualities on the one hand, and the theory of the four humors with their temperaments on the other, a system of pharmacology was evolved in which individual drugs could

```
LIVER                    hot                    HEART
   yellow bile                                 blood
      (choleric)                            (sanguine)


              FIRE    │   AIR
  dry ───────────────────┼───────────────────── moist
              EARTH   │   WATER


      (melancholic)   │        (phlegmatic)
      black bile      │           phlegm
  SPLEEN             cold              BRAIN
```

be mixed as indicated by their primary qualities.

Unlike what we find in Indian thought, Greek philosophy and science (at least until the time of Aristotle) regarded the reliability of the senses as by no means self-evident, and there was a reluctance to link the primary qualities regarded as properties of the elements with the corresponding sensory perceptions. To the best of my knowledge, this discrepancy between theory and sensory perception has never appeared in Indian philosophy and science.

By combining the doctrine of the primordial elements with the idea that their sensory perception is possible, Galen succeeded in devising a pharmacology similar to the *Dravyaguna*. For the first time in Europe, the sense of taste was recognized as an instrument for detecting the primary qualities. Setting out from the tastes, the effects of medicinal plants in or on the body were empirically observed, and the dominance of one or another of the primary qualities was inferred.

Galen mentions other senses, but the bulk of his fourth book is devoted to the sense of taste. He speaks of nine different tastes, adding to the six in the Ayurveda the tastes fatty and biting, and distinguishing between astringent and harsh.

17

PLANTS AND TASTES
The Vindication of the Senses

Admittedly, the classification of plants by their tastes is not sufficient or perfect. The isolation of the active principles of plants by modern methods of chemical analysis is an undeniable advance. But, when payment for this advance is made by sacrificing the holistic view, the price appears (to me, anyway) to be unacceptably high. If, being aware of this gain, we think we can dispense with 'tasting' our environment because we are now in possession of the exact chemical analyses of the impurities in our air and water and so on, it seems to me that we have already lost a part of our awareness. And if this gain causes our faith in the specific action of synthetic preparations to assume an almost sacramental character in spite of the growing list of drug-induced side effects, then we are acting against what should be our better judgment and are doing ourselves an unnecessary injury.

In order to redress the balance somewhat, I shall now describe certain medicinal plants in terms of their tastes and, in succeeding chapters, give numerous examples of plants under each taste. To some extent, I adopt the divisions of the classical texts, in particular the *Charaka Samhita*. But, since these describe mainly tropical and subtropical plants, I have also made the attempt—and, so far as I know, this is the first time anyone has done so—to categorize Central European plants by their tastes according to Ayurvedic criteria, carefully checking my own personal experience against the plant taste descriptions found in herbals.

However, I am not pretending to offer a complete scheme or listing. For one thing, my aim is to give practical examples that will encourage the reader to make direct contact with nature for himself or herself and to trust his or her own senses when 'communicating' with plants.

I have been particularly interested in seeing to what extent the Ayurvedic system could be transferred to Europe. The more I have familiarized myself with the material, the greater has been my astonishment at the success of the transfer. It goes without saying that there were doubtful points requiring elucidation from my Indian teachers, and the response to this book may help to clear up other difficulties.

The time has now come to issue a serious warning. On no account should the reader start eating or even tasting unfamilair leaves, fruits, or roots. It is essential to be very cautious and to come to terms with this centuries-old and long-neglected knowledge slowly and painstakingly. We have to attend the 'primary school of the senses' again, and need to work hard at the subject before we can presume to judge the medicinal contents and uses of a plant from its appearance and taste. There are a number of extremely poisonous plants about, so please, *never take foolish risks—taste nothing unless you are absolutely certain it is edible and harmless.* Remember, too, that every system has its exceptions.

An immediate advantage, however, is a better appreciation of the role of taste in our daily diet. (By diet I mean any intake of food that is appetizing, health giving, and suitable to the needs of the individual.) In this context, it goes without saying that we ourselves are responsible for eating nourishing, safely processed food items of known origin and avoiding synthetic products and items which are heavily laced with chemicals. Perhaps this is easier said than done, but even in the industrialized countries there is a trend toward supplying uncontaminated, organically grown produce.

18

THE SWEET LIFE

The Taste Madhura, *with Examples of Its Action*

Madhura, the sweet taste, imparts recognizable qualities to food. It is pleasant, mild, and slightly greasy, and brings about a change in the consistency of the saliva. In the language of chemical analysis, sugars, carbohydrates, fats, and amino acids all have this taste. Sweet is composed of the elements earth (*Prthivi*) and water (*Jala*), and its *Gunas* or properties are heavy (*guru*), cold (*sita*), oily (*snigdha*), and gelatinous (*picchila*).

The action of this taste on the three *Doshas* is to increase *Kapha* and make it ebullient, and to reduce *Vata* and *Pitta*. On the *Dhatus* its action is anabolic, and it promotes tissue building and the life of the body elements. Because of its heavy quality, its effect on *Agni*, the digestive fire, is to slow down the processes of digestion. Its oily and gelatinous nature give it a blocking (constipating) effect on the ducts.

However we choose to picture a piece of cake in our imaginations, the above basic description is what sweetness means to Ayurveda. A quick lick with the tongue supplies the key to its working in the whole body.

However, the general effect of sweet can be stated even more exactly than this. The sweet taste strengthens the memory, reduces the risk of abortion, helps against burning sensations and thirst, promotes lactation (milk secretion), and acts as an antitoxin. Sweet operates as a tonic if the digestion is working normally and the ducts of the body, the *Srotas*, are open. If this is not the case, pungent and bitter substances must be taken first in order to regulate the digestion and to clean out the canals.

In therapy sweet is employed for general debility and where there is a danger of miscarriage, and to help the female to secrete milk and the male to produce semen. It is used, therefore, when there is an increase in *Vata* and *Pitta*.

Contraindications are all those diseases which are caused by an excess of *Kapha*, for example, obesity and colds or chills.

An excessive intake of sweet things causes a whole series of diseases, from obesity (of course) to ponderousness, loss of appetite, and depression. The chance of catching cold is increased, and coughs and sneezes, asthma, fever, and indigestion are further signs that the balance of the tastes is not being kept in the meals and that too many sweet things are being eaten. Lymphadenitis, conjunctivitis, and tumors all belong to the list of diseases that can be caused by an excess of sweet.

Sweet is the prevailing taste in practically all our staple foods such as wheat, barley, rye oats, millet, maize, and rice. Plants like the potato, sweet potato, manioc (otherwise known as tapioca), sago, taro, and yam also belong to this group. Here we have the basic diets of all the peoples of the world, and each item is predominantly sweet. They share the way in which their fundamental elements are put together as well as the quality 'heavy', and they build up the tissues and provide energy.

An important group of foodstuffs with a mainly sweet flavor is that of the various oils such as sesame seed, peanut, coconut, sunflower seed, olive, and so on. Also, nuts like walnut, peanut, coconut, edible chestnut, etc., belong to the group of sweet foodstuffs, as of course do the sugars obtained from cane, beet, maple, and palm, together with all sweet fruits (even though the latter always have a sour after-taste). Finally, milk, sweet milk products, and flesh foods belong to the sweet-tasting group.

There are, however, important exceptions, namely honey and all legumes. The concept 'sweet as honey' is thought to be misleading by Ayurvedic theorists, who regard honey as principally astringent in character and appeal to the fact that it does not increase *Kapha* and is weight-reducing, unlike other items we call sweet.

Legumes do have a high protein content and are the most important providers of protein in the Indian kitchen, but they reinforce *Vata*. People with a dominant *Vata* factor in their makeups should eat few legumes.

Wheat (*Triticum vulgare Vill.—Gramineae*) is one of the oldest of cultivated plants. It originated in Western Asia. In Northern India it is more important than rice as a source of nourishment, and in Europe it is the staff of life practically everywhere. But we suffer a grievous loss when we purchase white, chemically bleached, lifeless, wrapped bread deprived of its vitamins, minerals, and bran. We ought to prefer the natural product freshly baked from organically grown grain because only then can wheat serve us both as food and medicine.

Wheat embryo, which is especially rich in vitamins, protein, oils, and mineral salts, can overcome debility, depression, heart and stomach disorders, and skin eruptions (rashes). It helps to calm *Vata* and to strengthen *Kapha*.

Wheatbran is very useful for removing harmful waste from the intestines and, by cleansing the bowels, tranquillizes all three *Doshas*. A wheat-bran bath will soothe inflamed and irritated skin—a *Pitta* disease.

Wheat gruel helps to relieve heartburn, eructation, stomach upset, colitis, and stomach and bowel cramps.

An excellent remedy for *Vata* diseases is oats (*Avena sativa L.—Gramineae*) It fortifies the system in young and old and strengthens the brain and nerves. Oat-straw baths are good for gout, rheumatism, lumbago, and liver complaints. Oatmeal gruel is an excellent 'spare diet' in disorders of the stomach and bowels. It strengthens *Kapha* and reduces *Vata* and *Pitta* and cures *Vata* and *Pitta* diseases.

Barley (*Hordeum vulgare L.*), too, has the characteristic mealy, sweet taste of the *Gramineae*. It reaches our tables chiefly in the form of (specially milled) pot barley. Barley gruel is a good diet for gastrointestinal troubles. Barley flour cooked in milk stimulates lactation.

Malt, which is barley prepared for brewing, helps to strengthen the body and is also employed as an expectorant.

One cereal that has almost been forgotten is millet (*Panicum miliaceum L.*), and yet a diet of millet is especially useful for restoring the intestinal flora after a course of antibiotics.

Like wheat, rye (*Secale cereale L.*) plays an important role. It will withstand a bleak climate and grows successfully in poor-quality soil. Its nutritious value is similar to that of wheat; although it contains less protein it is richer in mineral salts. Therefore, it is recommended for older people who are beginning to suffer from arteriosclerosis (hardening of the arteries).

The staple diet of the Indians is maize (*Zea mays L.*), which has spread over a great part of the world. Like wheat-germ oil, maize-germ oil contains many important vitamins and anabolic agents. Maize flour is used as a nutritious article in the diet.

Sali (*Oryza sativa L.—Gramineae*), or rice, is the staple diet of at least one third of the world's peoples. It is one of the oldest cultivated plants in the tropics, and it spread to Mediterranean countries as a consequence of the campaigns of Alexander the Great. There are different varieties of rice; the two most used are upland rice and rice that is grown on submerged land. The latter, owing to its special requirements, has had a formative influence on all Asiatic cultures and has encouraged tolerant behaviour. A mountain stream irrigates many terraces, and all the families in a village, or even all the villages in a district, are obliged to cooperate with one another in order to gather the crop safely. Feuds would endanger the harvest and would raise the specter of starvation. Therefore, the laws relating to water are very carefully drafted, and relationships between neighbors are nicely regulated.

For rice to retain its full nutritional value, it must be unpolished and retain its silver husk. Then it will act positively on all three *Doshas* and will be sweet, cooling, diuretic, beneficial to the eyesight, strengthening, and a tonic to the heart. Only those with stomach ulcers and diabetes should avoid it.

Another medicinal plant in the 'sweet group' is couch grass (*Agropyron repens L.–Gramineae*). Couch grass is related to wheat, but to the farmer it is nothing but a troublesome weed with a long creeping root. Troublesome or not, however, this sweet and slimy tasting root is found to be diuretic and blood purifying, and so it is helpful in the treatment of disorders of the liver and gall bladder as well as of the kidneys and bladder.

Certain plants such as the wild mallow (*Malva silvestris L.– Malvaceae*) manufacture a gummy substance which can be employed to coat raw or irritated surfaces and thus suppresses the overactivity of *Pitta* and *Vata*. The mallow is an age-old healing plant and is used both internally and externally in inflammations because of its soothing and emollient properties.

Marshmallow (*Althea officinalis*) belongs to the same family. Its alternative name, Bismalva (meaning twice as effective as ordinary mallow), has been given because of its stronger action. Its main application is in inflammations of the skin and mucous membranes. Marshmallow root tea is useful in inflammations of the bladder and uterus and in diarrhea, pyorrhea, furuncle, and a cough.

Similar in action is mullein (*Verbascum thapsus L.–Scrophulariaceae*). This plant, too, is soothing and emollient. A tea made from the flowers helps to break up phlegm in the chest and to relieve coughs. It brings relief in inflammation of the bladder and is blood purifying, diuretic, and tranquilizing.

The classical Sanskrit texts mention a number of effective herbal remedies classified under the taste 'sweet.' Here we can do no more than describe the most important and interesting. For example, there is a small, thorny, erect bush with long branches and little yellow flowers known as *Bala* (*Sida cordifolia L.–Malvaceae*). It grows only in damp clearings in the tropical and subtropical areas of India. Its root has great healing power in *Vata* diseases.

The *Bala* root is a *Rasayana* medicine, which means that it is rejuvenating. It is given as a tonic in the form of *Bala arista, arista* being the general term for a fermented decoction. To make it, the root is chopped up into very small pieces which are boiled in water. The resulting liquid is then filtered, and the filtrate is mixed with treacle in the ratio of 40 to 60, certain blossoms such as those of the *Woodfordia fructicosa* being added to assist fermentation. A container is then half-filled with the mixture, and is buried in the earth to keep it (as far as possible) at an even temperature, between 36 and 40 degrees Centigrade. Fermentation is complete at the end of about two months. Further ingredients are added to the syrup, the usual composition of the additive being long pepper, cinnamon, and cloves. This classic process, although it might try a European's patience, can also be used by ourselves—for example, in making ribwort syrup in the traditional style.

For the treatment of fevers, the Bala root is mixed with ginger. And in South India, Bala Taila, an oleaginous preparation, is a great favorite, being used for enemas and massage.

Taila is sesame oil, but the word can be used for any kind of oil. Coconut oil and peanut oil are common substitutes for sesame oil. Mustard oil, sandalwood oil, castor oil, beeswax and various fats are also used for specific oily preparations important in therapy. Oils, fats, and ghee (clarified butter) act not only as preservatives but as *Vata shamana*, i.e., they mitigate excessive *Vata*. Ghee—one of the most prized substances in the Indian kitchen—also acts as *Pitta shamana* and *Kapha shamana*, which means it affects all the *Doshas*. In the preparation of oils, the expressed juice or watery extract of the medicinal plant is mixed with the oil, and the water is then evaporated by slow heating.

Vidari (*Ipomea paniculata R. Br.—Convolvulaceae*) is a root known to be *Rasayana*, and it is used in powdered form as a tonic to relieve *Vata* and *Pitta* disorders.

Pancha trina mula is a blend of the roots of five different grasses: *Iksu*, the sugarcane (*Saccharum officinarum L.*); *Darbha* (*Imperata cylindrica Beauv.*); *Kusa* (*Demostachy bipinata*); *Kasa* (*Saccharum spontaneum L.*); and *Sali*, rice (*Oryza sativa L.*). This mixture of roots promotes milk secretion, is cooling and diuretic, and corrects disorders of the kidneys and bladder.

Another mixture, a very potent one compounded of ten different roots and known as *Dasa mula*, has a predominately astringent taste and so will be mentioned again in the appropriate chapter, but one of the roots is sweet and belongs to a herb conspicuous for its prominent woody-looking leaf veins: *Salaparni* (*Desmodium gangeticum Dc.–Leguminosae*). In fact, the name *Salaparni* means 'woody-leaf plant', from *sala* 'wood' and *parni*, 'leaf'. Its roots are a febrifuge and expectorant and are very effective in diarrhea.

Another important medicinal plant is *Gamhara* (*Gmelina arborea L.–Verbenaceae*), with a sweetish and slightly bitter fruit which helps to regenerate the tissues. The root cortex has an astringent taste and belongs to the *Dasa mula*.

Yastimadhu (*Glycyrrhiza glabra L.–Leguminosae*) is known to us as liquorice. Its sweet taste is accompanied by a slightly bitter flavor. Liquorice is an expectorant and also inhibits inflammation, especially in the case of gastritis and gastric ulcers. It has been used with more caution since it was found to contain a principle similar to cortisone. The classical texts credit it with an amazing power to strengthen the memory. The effect on the *Doshas Vata* and *Pitta* is calming.

A prized medicinal root, widely distributed in the ancient world and still well-known today, is that of asparagus. In India the sweet and somewhat bitter-tasting root *Satavari* (*Asparagus racemosus Will D.–Liliaceae*) is employed as a brain and nerve tonic. It is an appetizer, stimulates the breasts to secrete milk, helps to clear phlegm from the breathing passages, and has even managed to retain its reputation as an aphrodisiac.

Here in the West we cultivate *Asparagus officinalis*, the shoots of which are cut in spring and served as a vegetable. Unlike them the shoots contain no sugar but are a splendid article of diet for those suffering from kidney disease, for diabetics, and for convalescents. Like asparagus, the vine prefers a temperate climate. *Draksa*, the sweet grape (*Vitis vinifera L.–Vitaceae*), is a particularly valuable tonic. In India grapes are prepared as a fermented decoction, *Draksa arista*, which is good for disorders of the respiratory organs and improves the general resistance of the body. The purifying and decongestant action of this grape decoction on the lungs and breathing passages can be explained by the close embryonic relationship of the lungs and the gastrointestinal canal.

A sweet, energy-giving fruit—one of the main articles of diet among the Arabs—is the date, *Khajura* (*Phoenix sylvestris Roxb.–Palmae*). Ripe dates are a precious fruit with many virtues. They are delicious, rich, and nourishing, very digestible, and mildly aperient. The classical texts assure us that they encourage sperm production and also (and this is of tremendous benefit in a hot climate) that they prevent an excess of *Pitta*.

The coconut palm, *Kolpa Vriksa* (*Cocos nucifera* L.), is called in India 'the tree of heaven,' and with good reason, for every part of this plant has its value. 'We have nine hundred and ninety-nine uses for the tree of heaven,' says one Indian proverb. The fibers of the coconut and the leaves and the trunk of the palm are used as building materials. The coconut kernels, known as copra (from the Sanskrit *Khorpara*), are an important source of food and oil. Toddy, or palm wine, is obtained from the sugary juice of the bud tips.

The chief medicinal product of this palm is the milk of tender coconuts before they are fully ripe. It is cooling, aperient, and diuretic and is a splendid remedy for heartburn. Because of its nutritious and diuretic properties, it is prescribed in kidney diseases, and it is also an important item in the diet of patients suffering from subcutaneous dropsy, since it has a depletive action. Coconut milk is also an excellent remedy in fever, nausea, and cardiac insufficiency.

Our most important source of sugar is the sugarcane, *Iksu* (*Saccharum officinarum* L.—*Gramineae*). With its bright silver-grey tassels, it bears some resemblance to a reed. However, the stalk is not hollow but has a sweet pith containing approximately 15 percent sugar, and more still in the lower section of the stalk. The *Iksu* juice sellers are a familiar street sight in many parts of India; they work hard at pushing pieces of cane up to two meters long through rolling presses to extract the juice.

The sugarcane is grown within a relatively broad band on either side of the equator. The original home of the plant is South east Asia and the Pacific islands. In the wake of the conquests of Alexander the Great (during the period BC 334-324), the countries bordering the Mediterranean first heard tell of yet another wonder of the mysterious Indies: a 'solid honey not made by bees.' Until this point, sweetness had been associated in Europe and in much of the rest of the world only with fruit and honey. The 'new' sugar was at first a costly imported item reserved for the tables of princes. Then, between the seventh and ninth centuries, the Arabs introduced sugarcane into the Mediterranean region and, later on, after the discovery of America, the plant was taken to Mexico and Brazil and to what were to become the new 'sugar islands,' Cuba and Jamaica.

By its mild diuretic and aperient action, sugar promotes the excretion of waste products. Those suffering from kidney disease can take larger amounts of sugar, because it is easily digested and is proteinfree. The same goes for those infected with hepatitis since the recourse to sugar offers some measure of protection to liver cells unable to tolerate fats or proteins during this illness. (Incidentally, it is interesting to note that by serving sweets toward the end of a meal we acknowledge the old truth that sweet things help to take the edge off the appetite.)

The most important animal product in India is *ghee*. Ghee is made from butter heated to a medium temperature. The froth is skimmed off several times, and the substance is then allowed to cool a little and, after the removal of the skin, it is strained very slowly through a fine sieve so that the sediment is left behind. In this way all the solid components are removed, and the ghee will no longer turn rancid. If need be (and many classical recipes are based on this property), it will keep for a hundred years.

The best ghee comes from cow's milk; it is sweet and strengthening, aids digestion, promotes sperm production, strengthens *Ojas* and the energy field surrounding an individual, and also increases *Meda Dhatu* and the *Dosha Kapha*. It preserves the eyesight, helps in cases of galloping consumption and in poisonings, and enjoys a reputation as an aphrodisiac. This ghee also cures mental disturbances caused by disharmonies of the three *Doshas*, and acts quite powerfully on the mind—it improves the memory and stabilizes the intellect, and reduces overactivity in *Vata*, *Pitta*, and *Kapha*.

Ghee prepared from goat's milk is strengthening too, and it sharpens the appetite and improves the eyesight. It is useful in bronchitis, asthma, and tuberculosis, and is easily digested. The product of digestion disperses an excess of *Kapha*. Ghee from sheep's milk is very digestible. It does not stimulate *Pitta*, and it counteracts increased and agitated *Kapha* and *Vata* and helps in trembling, edema, and female diseases. Mare's milk ghee stimulates the digestion and pacifies Kapha. Ghee from human milk strengthens the body, is easily digested, improves the eyesight, and acts as an antidote against poisons.

The longer ghee is kept the more valuable it becomes. Old ghee cures gray cataract, chronic nasal catarrh, asthma, bronchitis, vertigo, epilepsy, refractory skin diseases, poisonings, colicky pains in the female genital tract, diseases of the eyes and ears, swellings, and fevers. It is also an excellent treatment in mental derangement and for purifying and healing ulcers. It regulates the bowels and calms all three *Doshas*. Ten-year-old ghee is a tonic and is an efficacious remedy for fever. Ghee that is older still is strongly rejuvenating. The old manuscripts inform us that hundred-year-old ghee can cure all diseases caused by *Rakshasas*, i.e., demons.

In contrast to ghee, butter plays a very subordinate role in India. Fresh butter is mainly sweet but is also slightly astringent and acidic due to traces of buttermilk. Butter is said to be aphrodisiac and energy giving, and it stokes up the digestive fire and increases sperm production; it also calms overexcited *Vata* and *Pitta* and those states of mind in which, as we say, 'the blood boils.' It is beneficial in pulmonary consumption, hemorrhoids (piles), facial palsy, bronchitis, and emaciation, and is prescribed for enlargement of the spleen, disorders of the brain, swellings, and lethargy. Stale butter is alkaline, pungent and sour, makes the eater vomit, and causes hemorrhoids and obstinate skin diseases; it increases *Kapha*, is heavy, and makes body fat.

Milk itself is a fundamental article of diet with good therapeutic properties. It is sweet, heavy, fat, and cooling. Medically, it is aperient, generally strengthening, tranquillizing, and an improver of the appetite. Ayurveda uses human milk and milk from various animals such as cows, goats, sheep, camels, water buffaloes, mares, and elephants. Milk from all these sources contains the essence, the *Rasa*, of many medicinal plants and is therefore a life giver. The place where the animals graze influences the milk's consistency. From the lush upland meadows comes the richest and heaviest milk; low-lying, waterlogged, or parched fields afford light, less creamy milk.

Milk is particularly good for children and the elderly, for the thin and weak, and for those who are convalescing from a fever. It is also recommended for those whose digestive fire is too fierce. Generally speaking, milk allays the sensation of heat generated by food and drink taken during the day; for this reason the ancient texts advise us to drink milk at night. What we should at all costs avoid, however, is to drink milk with salt or sour foods, as doing so could result in skin diseases. The classics also point out the effects of certain containers on the properties of milk. Milk out of a copper vessel calms *Vata*, out of a gold vessel calms *Pitta*, out of a silver bowl calms *Kapha*, and out of a brass vessel helps to make blood.

The milking time is significant, too. During the day the animals actively forage for fresh vegetation. Evening milk is very wholesome and assuages and reduces all three *Doshas*. Morning milk is cold and thick and causes lassitude and drowsiness; it makes a person dull and increases *Kapha*.

The milk from different animals also differs in effect. Cow's milk is sweet and at the same time astringent. It is light, rejuvenating, and strenghening, is a heart tonic and, because it strengthens the intellect and the vital powers, is spoken of in the old texts as an elixir of life. It has a reducing action on all three *Doshas*, but especially on *Pitta* (provided, of course, that it is fresh, warm cow's milk, since cold milk can upset the *Doshas* even when it reduces *Pitta* a little). It is useful in consumption of the lungs, vertigo, coughs, fever, and diarrhea. The classical texts even go so far as to distinguish the effects of milk from different colored cows. Milk from black cows is said to be of the highest quality; it reduces *Vata*. Milk from yellow cows reduces *Pitta* and *Vata*, milk from white cows agitates *Kapha*, and milk from red cows agitates *Vata*.

Goat's milk is much prized in the Ayurvedic texts. Infants for whom human milk is not available should be fed on goat's milk. Goats are lean animals; in the main they eat pungent and bitter herbs and drink little water. They are very agile and are always on the move. All these qualities are imparted to their product. Goat's milk is astringent and sweet, light and cooling, and constipating. It is recommended in diarrhea, tuberculosis, bronchitis, fever, and hemorrhages. Goat's milk, when boiled and allowed to cool, reduces *Vata* and *Pitta* if drunk in the morning.

Sheep's milk is sweet, fat, and heavy. It is especially good for patients suffering from disturbed *Vata*, and relieves bronchitis and gout. Sheep's milk ought always to be boiled and should be drunk while still hot.

Mare's milk is strengthening and heals *Vata* diseases of the limbs. It is not very fat. The main taste is sweet and sour, and the *Anurasa*, or fugitive flavor, is salty and pungent.

Human milk is used as a medicine only when it is cold. It is digestible and fat, has a strengthening effect, and nourishes the seven *Dhatus*. The mother who is supplying the milk should not eat anything that is too pungent, sour, salty, astringent, or alkaline.

Flesh foods, too, have a mainly sweet taste; they supply energy but tend to lie heavily on the stomach. Meat soup, on the other hand, is very easily digested. Most Indians are vegetarians, Moslems and Christians being exceptions to the rule. Nevertheless, the therapeutic character of animal foods is accurately described in the Ayurvedic texts, which place them in two distinct classes according to the habitats of the animals concerned. The flesh of animals living in *Jangala* terrain is quite different from that of animals living in *Anupana* terrain.

Jangala terrain is an arid waste high in the mountains, with little water and, in general, no pools or marshes. In other words, it is an expression of *Vata*. The large group of animals found there is divided into eight subgroups; examples are animals that live in burrows or caves. Domestic animals occupy another subgroup. Usually, the flesh of these creatures is sweet and rather astringent; it is lean and light, energy giving, and stimulating to the appetite. It regulates all three *Doshas* and has a curative action on speech disorders, facial palsy, deafness, nausea, chronic heart disease, and diabetes. The frequency here of diseases implying a disturbed (and usually reduced) *Vata* is quite interesting.

Anupana terrain is characterized by the presence of water in the form of humidity, luxuriant vegetation, and rain forests, things mostly associated with *Kapha*. The subgroups of animals found in it include those living near water, swimmers, fish, etc. *Anupana* flesh is sweet, fat, and heavy. It reduces the digestive fire and helps to regulate *Kapha*, but it tends to block the *Srotas* and is suitable only when the digestion is sound.

19

WHEN WE TURN SOUR

The Taste Amla, *with Examples of Its Action*

Amla, the sour taste, participates in the elements earth and fire, and its main properties are heavy, hot, and oily. Its sources of flavor are organic acids such as oxalic acid and the fruit acids. Characteristic of this taste are a slight stinging in the mouth and throat and increased salivation. Acidic foods are diaphoretic, appetizing, and cleansing.

Sourness strengthens *Kapha* and *Pitta* but reduces *Vata*. Its action on the biological fire, *Agni*, is strengthening, and therefore aids digestion. In therapeutic use, it restores the balance of overemphasized *Vata* and corrects digestive disorders and loss of appetite. Contraindications are disturbances of *Pitta* and *Kapha* such as gastritis, internal bleeding, and jaundice. Overindulgence in sour things will encourage various diseases: it will upset the composition of the blood and will cause muscle weakness (myasthenia), dropsy, inflammations, and any illness caused by an increase of *Pitta*.

The largest group of sour food items is that of the fruits, some only when unripe but others even when ripe. It is common knowledge that fruits are important sources of vitamins. The classic Ayurvedic texts knew nothing of 'vitamins,' of course, yet they did have much to say about effects now associated with vitamins, and they emphasized the importance of sour foods in a balanced diet.

We often have occasion to refer to sourness in the things we eat, sometimes metaphorically as in the expression 'sour grapes,' and on occasion we even use the term when speaking of ourselves and exclaim, 'I feel sour today!' When that happens we are suffering from an excess of *amla*. Being overly sour cannot only produce *Pitta*-type diseases in the body, but it can disturb the mind as well.

No one is astonished when told that the main taste of the gooseberry is *amla*, but it may be rather surprising to learn that 'sweet' berries like the raspberry and currant are included in the *amla* group and have the super-added taste *madhura* only when ripe.

The mango, *Amara* (*Mangifera indica L.–Anacardiaceae*) is one of the best-known and most-loved fruits in the tropics. The original home of the mango tree is in Burma, Assam, and Malaysia. Under the Moguls, and later through the Portuguese, the plant was introduced into other tropical regions. Portuguese monks, in fact, cultivated the choicest variety, 'Alfonso.' The tree, which can grow to a height of thirty meters, spreads its branches to cast a refreshing shade, and bears cream-colored, scented panicles. Yet of the thousands of individual blossoms, only relatively few produce the ripe fruit, which hangs down on long stalks. In the middle of the fibrous pulp there is a very large kernel enclosing the embryo. The fruit has a sweet and sour flavor.

In the tropics, the mango is a staple article of diet. Ayurveda recommends the fruit for the elderly with weak constitutions who are suffering from an excess of *Vata*. The mango soothes inflammations of the colon (colitis) and improves the complexion.

From Iran comes the pomegranate, *Dadima* (*Punica granatum L.–Punicaceae*). The Latin term *granatum* was chosen because the seeds look like semiprecious stones. The tree grows to as much as five meters high and has tough and occasionally thorny branches. The fruit swells to a diameter of up to nine centimeters, has a leathery reddish-yellow skin, and a red, sweet-and-sour pulp packed full of seeds. There are various kinds of pomegranate, some sweeter some sourer. Sour pomegranates increase the flow of saliva and gastric juice. The juice squeezed from the sweeter varieties is a favorite cooling and nutritious drink and is good for bleeding gums.

What is as sharp as a lemon? The important group of citrus fruits extends its range from the tropics to the subtropics and is a well-known source of vitamins. The most widely distributed fruit in this group is the lime (*Citrus aurantifolia L.–Rutaceae*), an oval fruit not more than six centimeters across, and closely related to the lemon and frequently found in India and Southeast Asia. The branches of the tree are set with thorns, the leaves have winged stipules, and the white flowers are heavily scented. Unlike the more Mediterranean lemon, the lime does not yellow as it ripens but remains green. Its juice stimulates the flow of saliva and gastric juice, relieves flatulence, nausea, and cramps, is cooling in fevers and sunstroke, and brings chronic diarrhea under control.

The lemon is another of those Eastern products that came to the Mediterranean regions in the wake of the conquests of Alexander the Great and, once there, spread rapidly. As a source of vitamin C the lemon is a splendid preservative of health even when—due to bad weather, seasonal change, or epidemic—external conditions are unfavorable.

Synthetic vitamin C is not a perfect substitute for the action of the lemon whatever the pharmaceutical industry may say to the contrary. When people engage in technical discussions of this contentious issue, an important aspect of the case is often ignored. They concentrate on the chemical structures of the end-products in typical Western fashion, and pay scant attention to the differences in the production processes. But surely we ought to attach some importance to the disparity between what goes on in a chemical factory that pollutes the environment and the gentle reactions in a living, fragrant orange or lemon tree? It might make sense, as far as useful synthetic drugs are concerned, to confine ourselves to those not made by plants.

Lemon juice, mixed with a pinch of salt, allays nausea, vomiting, and digestive disorders. Mixed with honey and a sprinkling of black pepper, it cures hiccups and heartburn caused by gas generated in the digestive tract. At the Ayurvedic Hospital in Benares, patients with infectious hepatitis are treated with nothing but lemon juice and glucose.

In Europe the hips or fruit of the dog rose (*Rosa Canina L.—Rosaceae*) are highly prized for their vitamin C content. Usually the hips are dried and are prepared as a tea, but a delicious jam can be made from the fruit after the seeds have been removed, and this forms an excellent source of vitamin C for the dark and stressful winter months.

The juice of the orange-colored fruit of the sea buckthorn (*Hippophae rhamnoides L.—Elaeagnaceae*) helps in debility and influenza, restores the appetite, and makes good deficiencies in the elderly.

The juice of the raspberry (*Rubus idaeus L.—Rosaceae*) is aperient, appetizing, blood purifying, diuretic, diaphoretic, and generally refreshing and strengthening—we are referring to the fresh juice, of course. Raspberry syrup is employed to make unpleasant medicines more palatable.

Some sour plants contain an acid known as oxalic acid. Such plants should be eaten sparingly when raw. The best known example is the sorrel (*Rumex acetosa L.—Polygonaceae*). Sorrel is refreshing, blood purifying, appetizing, and digestive. Cooking greatly reduces its oxalic acid content.

Wood sorrel or shamrock, which is a European folk remedy as well as an entry in the Ayurvedic pharmacopoeia, contains oxalic acid, too. The herb must be used only when fresh. The infusion makes a refreshing, blood purifying, and diuretic drink. Ayurveda recommends the juice of the wood sorrel, *Cangeri* (*Oxalis acetosella L.—Oxalidaceae*), in cancerous tumors and in shaking palsy.* It is used both internally and externally.

The pods of the tamarind, *Amlika (Tamarindus indica L.— Leguminosae)*, are much used. The twenty-five meter high tree has a very thick top. It is often found fringing subtropical streets to provide shade. The slightly curved pods, eight to fifteen centimeters long, are green and sour when unripe and dark brown and sweetish-sour when ripe. Tamarind sold as 'fresh' is a half-dried, mangled, sticky mass of pods minus seeds. The fresh pulp juice, mixed with sugar and a pinch of salt, is dispensed for suntroke, fever, biliousness, and acute diarrhea, and is also an effective antidote for thorn apple poisoning and alcoholism. In Europe a tamarind conserve is employed as a mild laxative.

Amalaki (Emblica officinalis Gaertn.—Euphorbiaceae) is not a typical representative of *amla* because although its leading taste is sour it is also pungent, bitter, astringent, and sweet. Its potency (*Virya*) is cool and its aftertaste (*Vipaka*) is sweet. The tree is of medium height and bears small inconspicuous flowers and round greenish fruits two to three centimeters in diameter. *Amalaki* flourishes in the tropics and subtropics and is especially important as an ingredient in the *Tri Phala*, or 'Three Fruits', a predominantly astringent medicinal compound to be described in a following chapter. The fruit is eaten either fresh or dried. It strengthens the liver, is cooling and mildly laxative, and is beneficial in *Pitta* disorders. *Amalaki* is added to many tonics, probably because of its high vitamin C content. Dried *amalaki* fruit helps in diarrhea and dysentery.

Milk and yoghurt belong to the group of sour foods, and both form an important part of a typical Indian meal. Applied externally, yoghurt is good for nerve and joints pains.

---

* Translator's note: It hardly requires stressing that serious conditions such as these should be referred immediately to a qualified medical practitioner.

20

THE SALT OF LIFE

The Taste Lavana, *with Examples of Its Action*

Lavana, or saltiness, is a synthesis of the basic elements water and fire. Its leading properties are heavy, hot, oily (fatty), and pungent (sharp). The taste is carried by the various salts.

Minerals are very important for the function of all life systems. Without salt there would be no life. Salts are characterized by being easily soluble and hygroscopic (attracting moisture). Saltiness changes the consistency of the saliva, creates a burning sensation in the mouth and throat, softens the food, and puts an edge on the appetite. The salt taste stimulates the *Doshas Pitta* and *Kapha* and reduces *Vata*. The action on the *Dhatus* is catabolic (it assists the breaking down of the tissues).

The capacity of salts for retaining liquids can result in a physical sensation of laxness. Their effect on the *Malas* is aperient and diuretic, and they help to expel wind. They increase the digestive power of *Agni* and improve the appetite. As far as the *Srotas* are concerned, salt things clean the body's ducts because their hygroscopic action loosens tough plugs of matter and their pungency provokes expectoration.

In general, the salt taste is moistening and emetic and promotes salivation, digestion, and bowel motion. Salt remedies are given for loss of appetite and poor digestion and as an expectorant in coughs (also where *Vata* is in excess).

Contraindications are disturbed *Pitta*, skin complaints, swellings, high blood pressure, hemorrhages, and gastritis (inflammation of the lining of the stomach).

Too much salty food can cause a number of disorders, essentially the same as those brought about by an increase in *Pitta* or *Kapha*: thirst, loss of consciousness, fever, premature death of tissue cells, skin diseases, dropsy, odontoptosis (loose teeth), impotence, impaired functioning of the sense organs, premature gray hair, hair loss, gastritis, erysipelas, and eczema.

The above unfortunate consequences of a diet that is too rich in salt are all too common in the West. Industrialization has had a harmful effect to our eating habits. More and more salt is being consumed to compensate for the loss of taste in our standardized, preserved, denatured, and overcooked food. Even so, this compensation is not being made with carefully measured amounts of salt but according to the dictates of jaded palates. In Indian kitchens, salt is still used like any other condiment.

Ayurveda distinguishes between the different therapeutic actions of various salts:

Saindhava Lavana, or rock salt, is obtained from salt mines and is regarded as the salt with the best therapeutic effects. It usually contains other minerals such as iron and magnesium. Its color is white. It has a calming effect on all three *Doshas,* is light and fatty, strengthens the eyesight, and stimulates the digestion. It is also regarded as a heart tonic and aphrodisiac. One of its properties makes it exceptional as a salt: it is cooling although according to the general rule it ought to be heating. In India it is found mainly in the Indus region and in Sindh (from which it gets its name, *Saindh*). Rock salt has played a significant part in European history, too.

Samu, the sea, has given *Samudra Lavana,* or sea salt, its name. *Samudra* is obtained by the evaporation of sea water. Its color is white, it is fatty, and it has no pronounced aperient effect. *Samudra* is heavy and not particularly heating. One of its special properties is termed *avidahi* by the Indians, which means that it does not cause a burning sensation. In its action on the three *Doshas* it stimulates *Kapha* and calms *Vata.*

Sambhava or *Romaka Lavana* is the sodium carbonate and ammonium chloride found in barren alkaline soil. In India it is traditionally used for washing clothes. *Sambhava* has a dirty white color, is expectorant, diuretic, appetizing, digestive, and calming to *Vata.*

Bida and *Sauvarcala* are other kinds of rock salt. Both kinds are found in mines and are variously colored light red or dark red due to traces of other minerals. *Bida* rock salt contains sulphur, ammonium, and potassium and is mentioned in the *Charaka Samhita.* Charaka describes the manner in which salt was applied in his era: 'All these salts are fatty, hot and pungent and they increase the appetite to an exceptional degree. They are also used in embrocations, massage and thermotherapy, and as aperients and emetics, and to eliminate disturbed *Doshas* from the head region; in surgery they enter into the composition of dentifrices, suppositories, eye-drops and ointments. They are employed to treat digestive disorders and *Vata* diseases.'

The importance of salt is underlined by the fact that in nearly every country in the world trading in salt is a state monopoly. The British held the salt monopoly in India during the days of the Raj until Mahatma Gandhi led a demonstration to the seashore, scooped up some water, let it evoporate in the hot sun, and showed the white crystals covering his hands to the people milling round him; thus, at one stroke, the power of the monopoly was broken.

21

A Bit of 'Bite'

The Taste Katu, with Examples of Its Action

Katu, the pungent taste, is derived from the elements air and fire. Its basic properties are light, hot, and dry. Characteristic of this taste are a tingling sensation on the tongue, an increased flow of saliva, and sometimes lachrymation. The chief chemical vehicles of this taste are the essential oils.

Generally speaking, the action of the taste on the three *Doshas* is to strengthen *Vata* and *Pitta* and to reduce *Kapha*. Its action on the *Dhatus* is catabolic, absorptive, and drying. It strengthens *Agni* and therefore sharpens the appetite and promotes digestion. On the *srotas* it has a cleansing effect since its dryness absorbs liquids and brings about gentle expectoration.

Pungent items are usually reviving, cleanse the mouth and inhibit coagulation, stimulate the nerves, and are useful in digestive disorders and heart and skin complaints. In therapy, pungent things are given for loss of appetite and as a vermifuge, a dentifrice, a remedy for obesity and diabetes, and as a treatment for coughs, colds, asthma, and skin diseases.

This taste is indicated in disturbed and increased *Kapha* and in disturbed and reduced *Vata*.

Contraindications are disturbed *Pitta*, lack of urination, and faulty sperm production. An unbalanced diet containing an excess of pungent foods can cause a number of complaints: faintness, debility, impotence, giddiness, burning sensations, tremors, thirst, and nerve pain.

In European practice the etheric oils are used in the following ways:

1   External use: as a cutaneous stimulant—for example, oil of turpentine; to soothe pain and irritation—for example, peppermint oil and thyme oil; to allay inflammation—for example, camomile oil; as a disinfectant—for example, the oils of rosemary, peppermint, thyme, and carnation.

2   Internal use: as a condiment to sharpen the appetite and aid

digestion—for example, the oils of fennel, aniseed, and caraway; as an antispasmodic and anti-gripe remedy—for example, the oils of peppermint, camomile, fennel, coriander, peppergrass, or marjoram; as expectorants and stimulators of secretion which are also antispasmodic and antiseptic—for example, the oils of thyme, aniseed, and fennel; as a diuretic—for example, parsley and juniper oil; as cholagogues (agents to increase the flow of bile)—for example, the oils of peppermint and turpentine; as agents to increase the secretion of milk—for example, caraway and fennel oils. The flowers of the lime, elder, and camomile are diaphoretic (they promote perspiration). Thyme and tansy expel worms. Lemon balm, lavender, and valerian are tranquilizers.

3　Inhalants for diseases of the upper and lower air passages: the oils of peppermint, turpentine, and eucalyptus.

4　Corrigents of the senses of smell and taste: for example, peppermint, rose, and lavender oil.

When the diet has become one-sided, the balance needs to be restored in keeping with national eating habits. A foreigner suddenly introduced to Indian cooking might find that it is too pungent and that his digestion is being overstimulated. Climatic conditions in the subcontinent call for a particular combination of flavors which strike us as exotic but, to Indians, are refreshing, stimulating, and purifying.

Many aromatic plants are pungent and, being both aromatic and pungent, they increase the appetite so that meals are more enjoyable. By making the mouth water they assist the work of digestion. Not a few of these herbs also stimulate the membranes of the stomach and intestines to increase their production of digestive juices; this is especially useful when heavy meals are being consumed and when there is extra waste material to be eliminated fairly quickly. Other pungent aromatic plants influence lipid metabolism (the metabolism of fats and fatlike substances), reduce the cholesterol level, and help to prevent arteriosclerosis, myocardial infarction, and apoplexy.

According to the classical Ayurvedic texts, *Trikatu*, 'The three seasonings', is compounded of equal parts of ginger, long pepper, and black pepper, and is given in *Kapha* and *Vata* disorders.

Ginger (*Zingiber officinale Rosc.—Zingiberaceae*) has different Sanskrit names according to its preparation. Dried ginger is called *Sunthi*, and fresh ginger is called *Adraka*. The distinction is necessary because of a difference in properties. *Sunthi* is light and oily. *Adraka* is heavy, drying, and penetrating. Ginger is valued therapeutically for its warming effect, but its taste after digestion is sweet, with the result that ginger is the exception in its group and does not excite or strengthen *Pitta* but can be enjoyed by people in whom any of the three *Doshas* predominates.

The homeland of this herb is tropical Asia. When several years old, the plant has long leaves and thick, scaly, branching rhizomes. It bears purple-lipped yellow flowers. The fleshy root is used either fresh or dried, i.e., as *Adraka* or *Sunthi*. To dry them, the pieces are first boiled in water or milk, then simply left out in the sun. Ginger was brought to Europe by the Arabs quite early on, but it was the imperial British who were the first Westerners to give it a regular place in their kitchens. (They even turned it into ginger beer.)

The root strengthens the stomach, promotes the secretion of saliva, aids digestion, and is decongestant and antiinflammatory. Ayurveda recognizes many ways of using it. For example, when fresh ginger dressed with lemon juice and a pinch of salt is chewed fifteen minutes or so before a main meal, *Agni*, the digestive fire (and in fact all thirteen types of *Agni*—in the stomach, the liver, and the cells), is greatly energized.

A drink made of ginger paste and sugar boiled in milk makes a very effective domestic remedy for colds and chills. Dried ginger acts well in diets for the treatment of rheumatism and rheumatic carditis if the dose is gradually increased. Interesting, too, is the fact that ginger helps both in chronic diarrhea and in chronic constipation.

In India's hot and dry season, ginger is taken with sugar and ghee. In the rainy season it is taken with rock salt, and in the cold season it is taken with honey.

There is no doubt that the spice that has made the deepest mark on human history is pepper. It was already being mentioned as an Indian plant in the writings of Hippocrates. In the Middle Ages more value was placed on a sack of pepper than on a human life, and a common mode of telling someone to make himself scarce was to wish him in Pepperland! Pepper was, and still is, the most important spice on the world market. It was the most expensive commodity carried along the caravan routes, played a significant part in trade wars like the struggle for supremacy between Venice and Genoa, and was a prime economic motive in the search for a sea route to India. Its high price inevitably led to adulteration of the powdered form and, even today, it is advisable to buy the whole peppercorns.

Among the most important varieties are *Marica*, or black pepper (*Piper nigrum L.*) *Pippali*, or long pepper (*Piper longum L.*), and *Cavya*, or cubeb pepper (*Piper cubeba*). In India all three are used both for culinary and for medicinal purposes.

Whereas *Pippali*, the long pepper, is an insignificant looking creeping plant with a vertical root, *Marica*, the black pepper, is a lignified climbing plants with aerial roots, and like our European hops is grown on poles. Its broad, oval, shiny leaves have prominent longitudinal veins running from stalk to tip, and some fifty individual flowers are bunched together in each inflorescence. The round berries, approximately six millimeters in diameter, are picked shortly before they are ripe. Drying turns them into the familiar black pepper; when peeled, they are sold as white pepper.

Black pepper is 'dry;' therapeutically it is heating, and its digestive product is pungent. In general, pepper suits those who display the chracteristics of *Vata* and *Kapha* but not those with a predominance of *Pitta*.

Pepper sharpens the appetite and improves the digestion; it also helps to expel wind. The essential oil is secreted by the lungs and thus reduces discomfort in pharyngitis and tonsillitis. To treat these complaints, powdered pepper is mixed with honey and is taken three times a day. Powdered black pepper stirred into hot milk sweetened with sugar is used in bronchitis, for sore throats, and for headcolds. But note that only a pinch of pepper is used in these Indian household remedies.

Pastes and oils containing black pepper are used for rheumatism and skin diseases. A hot decoction of *Marica* (black pepper) is an effective mouthwash for toochaches.

Pepper is also sudorific and resembles quinine in its action. In fact, a mixture of pepper, ginger, and honey is prescribed for malaria. In small doses, *Piper cubeb* is given for disorders of the urinary passages. Long pepper is dispensed to children suffering from diarrhea, coughs, fever, and bronchitis; it is added to the diet of mothers to assist contraction of the uterus following delivery.

A particularly important plant in Ayurvedic therapy belonging to this tastegroup is *Chitraka* (*Plumbago ceylanica L.—Plumbaginaceae*), of which the ancient Sanskrit name was *Analanama*, from *Ana*, meaning 'fire.' This plant stimulates both the digestive fire and *Pachaka Pitta*. The taste of *Chitraka* is pungent both before and after digestion, its properties are light, dry, and keen, and its therapeutic action is heating.

Chitraka is a herb with white flowers and sticky oil glands. Only the knotty, reddish, dried root is used, mainly to aid digestion in *Vata* and *Kapha* diseases. Used externally, it raises blisters on the skin and forms part of the therapy in severe rheumatism.

Kustha, Indian Costus root (*Saussurea lappa C. B. Clarke—Compositae*) grows only in the high ranges of the Himalayas and in Kashmir; therefore this two-meter-high plant bearing large leaves and bluish-purple, nearly black flowers is also called *Kashmiri*. The brownish-yellow root is the part used; it has a characteristic strong odor, and its main taste is pungent with a touch of bitterness. The fundamental properties are light, dry, and rough, the therapeutic action is heating, and the taste after digestion is pungent. It is employed mainly in the treatment of coughs and asthma since it is expectorant and disinfectant, but it is also good in flatulence, skin disease, and in almost all *Kapha* disorders.

On descending to the jungle, we shall find a plant called *Vidanga* (*Embelia ribes—Myrsinaceae*), which is either a small tree or a large bush—it is difficult to tell which. It has oil glands in its leaves, bears tiny pale green flowers, and its round, reddish fruits are so small that they are commonly mistaken for seeds. Given with a laxative, these dried fruits are an excellent treatment for tapeworm. In addition to their *Prabhava* effect as a vermifuge, the small *Vidanga* fruits are good for flatulence and plethora because the taste and also the product of digestion are pungent, the properties are light, dry, and rough, and the therapeutic effect is heating.

From time immemorial, the Indian caste of launderers has been marking clothes with a pungent oil from the fruits of *Bhallataka*, the marking nut (*Semencarpus anacardium L. Anacardiaceae*); the fruits are known locally as 'elephant lice.' The effects of this East Indian plant place it in the pungent group even though, because the oil of the fruit blisters the skin, its pungency cannot be ascertained by tasting. Physicians, therefore, can utilize the fruits only after these have been treated to reduce their oil content. The fruits are mixed with small pieces of brick and are pounded in a cloth until completely pulverized. The crumbled brick, which absorbs all the plant oil, is flushed out at the end of the process. The treated fruit is good for hookworm, for *Vata* and *Kapha* diseases, and as *Rasayana*, or rejuvenating, medicine in old age.

Hingu, or stinking fennel (*Ferula narthex Boiss.—Umbelliferae*) was well-known to the Mediterranean peoples even in ancient times. An umbelliferous herb like fennel and dill, it is much used in Indian cooking. The gum resin prepared from its root, stem, and leaves is on sale in all the Indian markets and bazaars. Very characteristic is the strong scent (and taste) that suggested the plant's popular name. Its properties are light, viscous, quick, and mobile; its therapeutic action is heating, and its digestive product is pungent.

Hingu grows in Iran, Afghanistan, and the Indus region and is also found in wilderness and salt deserts. The resin has many outstanding qualities: it promotes digestion, expels wind, is disinfectant, antispasmodic, expectorant, and mildly aperient. Furthermore, it stimulates glandular secretion, improves the circulation, and strengthens the nerves.

The tall, tropical Indian lemon grass (*Cymbopogon Spec.—Gramineae*) does indeed have a very lemony smell. It tastes not only pungent but also bitter and even caustic. Its oil is utilized in making artificial lemon flavor. Taken in the form of a tisane (or tea), lemon grass is a febrifuge, diaphoretic and breaker of wind; it relieves stomach-ache and, when blended with sweet oils, is used as a rub for lumbago and rheumatism. In Europe lemon grass oil is sold mixed with balm oil. Carmelite spirits, or *Spiritus Melissae Compositus*, is a mixture of the oils of lemon, nutmeg, cinnamon, and carnation in alcohol.

Lemon balm (*Melissa officinalis L.—Lamiaceae*) is in Europe a favorite ingredient in herbal teas for settling the stomach, for expelling wind, and for promoting perspiration. But it is also employed as a tranquilizer in nervines. Externally the crushed fresh herb is used in compresses to treat abscesses and wounds that are not healing properly. Balm is also added to baths and to herb pillows for inducing sleep.

Rajika, or black mustard (*Brassica nigra L.—Brassicaceae*), produces pungent and slightly bitter seeds. In India, as formerly in Europe, mustard is employed as a popular remedy for abscesses and itching of the skin. Hot mustard plasters on the chest give relief from pains in the chest, coughs, bronchial catarrh, and shortness of breath. The warming effect is also beneficial in rheumatism and lumbago. Internally, mustard seed whets the appetite, expels worms, and is very helpful in *Vata* and *Kapha* disorders. Those who are characterized by a preponderance of *Pitta* should avoid it as they should avoid pungent things in general.

Quite similar to mustard in its medicinal properties is horseradish (*Armoracia rusticana G. M. et Sch.—Brassicaceae*). Mixed with honey, horseradish juice is a traditional gypsy remedy for bronchial complaints—and a very good one, too.

A species of basil which grows in nearly every Indian vegetable garden is *Tulsi*, or holy basil (*Ocimum sanctum L.—Lamiaceae*). It is offered in the temples and at household altars and releases a delightful carnationlike scent. Other types of basil, such as our European *Ocimum basilicum*, smell more of lemons or tarragon. Basil tea prepared from the leaves and flower heads is good for coughs and colds. The expressed juice, or a paste made from the bruised leaves, is given mixed with black pepper in malarial fever. The warm, pressed juice is used as eardrops and as a gargle in pharyngitis. It is also applied externally for skin complaints and insect bites.

Many *Kapha* diseases tend to raise the levels of fat and cholesterol in the blood. Very efficient prophylactics against this danger are several well-known kitchen herbs belonging to the *Lamiaceae* family: wild marjoram (*Origanum vulgare L.*), sweet marjoram (*Majorana hortensis Moench*), rosemary (*Rosmarinus officinalis L.*), and thyme (*Thymus vulgaris L.*). Wild marjoram expels pinworms and roundworms. Its leaves, when wrapped in a hot, wet cloth and used as a fomentation, are effective against the swellings, rheumatic pains, and colics caused by *Kapha* disorders. Marjoram tea is good for gripes and flatulence, for nasal catarrh, headache, and for calming the nerves. Thyme helps to prevent fermentation and putrefaction.

Jatiphala, the nutmeg (*Myristica fragrans Houtt—Myristicaceae*), comes from South India and is used in two forms: the seed itself, known as nutmeg, and the aril surrounding the seed, known as mace. Nutmeg expels wind, is astringent, is stimulating for poor circulation and low blood pressure, and (in higher doses) acts as an aphrodisiac. In whooping cough, embrocations of mace mixed with ghee are prescribed.

Garlic and onion have been known since ancient times, but are not, however, typical members of the pungent group since they also exhibit other strong flavors. Nevertheless, it is clear that the pungent taste is dominant in both plants, as may be seen from its effects.

Garlic (*Allium sativum L.—Liliaceae*) is called *Rasona* or 'one taste missing' in the old Sanskrit texts. *Rasona* possesses five of the six tastes: it is pungent, sweet, salty, bitter, and astringent. However, it is not sour; this is the missing flavor. Central Asia is the homeland of this culinary and medicinal herb. Its wide range of flavors makes it very versatile, and its properties are oily, keen, slimy, heavy, and mobile. It expels wind, loosens phlegm, is diuretic and antiseptic, inhibits the growth of bacteria, reduces the levels of fat and cholesterol, soothes inflammation, and acts as an aphrodisiac.

Palandu, the onion (*Allium cepa L.—Liliaceae*), is not used in medicine to the same extent that garlic is. In addition to its great pungency, it is noticeably sweet, and its digestive product is sweet, too. It is stimulating, diuretic, and expectorant.

A Westerner on a visit to India may take some time to become accustomed to the red patches etched everywhere into the asphalt streets and stone and plaster walls. These are the traces left by more than three hundred million people who are constantly chewing and expectorating betel. Betel chewing is an Indian passion. Shreds of betel nut mingled with a pellet of lime and aromatic herbs are rolled in a leaf from the betel vine and are then ready for mastication. The betel leaf (*Piper betle L.—Piperaceae*) is called in Sanskrit *Tambula* and in Hindi *Pan*, and comes from a climbing plant related to pepper. It contains a digestive enzyme, is a disinfectant, acts as a tonic in cardiac disorders, and is a regular ingredient in cough mixtures. The nut itself is from an entirely different plant and is, in fact, not a nut at all but a piece of dried seed from a certain palm (*Areca catechu*). The juice produced by chewing is generally stimulating and increases the flow of saliva—from which comes the above-mentioned discoloration of the streets.

But we have not yet come to the end of our pungent plants, among which are all the spices and aromatics. For example, aniseed (*Pimpinella anisum L.—Apiaceae*), fennel (*Foeniculum vulgare Mill.—Apiaceae*) and caraway (*Carum carvi L.—Apiaceae*) are valued as a warming seeds and are incorporated in many infusions taken for chest and stomach disorders. They are used as expectorants (to help clear the breathing passages of phlegm) and carminatives (to relieve the intestines of gas). Summer savory (*Satureia hortensis L.—Lamiaceae*), which has a peppery taste, is a popular seasoning. In addition to hindering putrefaction, removing phlegm, preventing spasms, and stimulating the digestion, it enlivens both body and mind. Garden chervil (*Anthriscus cerefolium L.—Apiaceae*), which tends to be displaced from vegetable patches by parsley (*Petroselinum crispum Mill.—Apiaceae*), is like the latter antiseptic, appetizing, a cholagogue (increasing the flow of bile), diuretic, and stimulating. Both plants inhibit milk secretion.

Hyssop (*Hyssopus officinalis L.—Lamiaceae*), dill (*Anethum graveolens L.—Apiaceae*), and lovage (*Levisticum officinale Koch—Apiaceae*), which are ordinary kitchen herbs, help to maintain health and have considerable remedial powers.

One of the most assertive examples of pungency is found in that type of paprika known as cayenne pepper or chilies (*Capsicum annuum L.—Solanaceae*). Tropical America is the original home of paprika. The Spaniards imported specimens of the plant to Europe, and in the seventeenth century the Portuguese introduced it into India and Indonesia. Today it would be unthinkable to find an Asiatic kitchen without this cheap, pungent seasoning so rich in vitamin C.

Now, although chilies taken in small amounts are appetizing, antiseptic, and an aid to digestion, larger amounts are dangerous and can injure the mucous membranes of the mouth and stomach. In Europe milder varieties of paprika are used, but these contain less vitamin C.

There is no space to extend our list of pungent plants indefinitely, but there is one very important plant that ought to be mentioned: camomile (*Matricaria chamomilla L.—Asteraceae*). It has a characteristic fragrance and taste and sedates all three *Doshas*; it is also antiseptic, antiphlogistic (antiinflammtory), antispasmodic, anodyne (soothing pain) and tranquilizing, and normalizes digestion and menstruation. The flowers are widely used in teas, gargles, and baths.

22

THE BITTER TRUTH
The Taste Tikta, with Examples of Its Action

The bitter taste *tikta* is derived from the elements air and ether. Its basic properties are light, cold, dry, and fine (or minute). Characteristic of bitter is that it eclipses all other flavors, reduces the flow of saliva, and makes the mouth dry. It also cleans the mouth and stimulates the appetite. The chemical vehicles of this taste are the bitters and various alkaloids and glycosides.

In its action on the *Tri Doshas*, bitter reinforces *Vata* and reduces *Pitta* and *Kapha*. In its action on the *Dhatus*, it is catabolic, absorptive, and drying. The bitter taste depletes *Meda*, the element of fat, *Mamsa*, the element of flesh, and *Majja* the element of marrow, and helps to counteract the pathogenic factors of diabetes. In acting on *Agni*, the digestive fire, bitter supports the *Vata* located in the stomach and small intestine by absorbing the mucus-producing *Kapha*. Bitter has a cleansing action on the body's ducts because its basic element air, and its inherent dryness, enable it to absorb slimy material, while its element ether naturally 'creates space', and its fineness or minuteness (or rather, power of penetration) gives it access to the finest branching channels.

The general effect of bitter is blood purifying and febrifuge. It removes suppuration, poisons, and wound secretions (serous exudations), and is a good remedy for skin diseases, poor appetite, and burning sensations.

Therapeutically, bitter-tasting things are employed in loss of appetite, digestive disorders, worms, gastritis, jaundice, skin diseases, fever, obesity, diabetes, and in increased secretions (whether purulent or serous).

Contraindications are disturbed *Vata* and lowered sperm production.

A whole of series of disorders can result from an unusually high intake of bitter foodstuffs: rawness of the ducts, symptoms of decay, physical weakness, dejection, sleepiness, and vertigo.

Increasing use is being made in Europe of bitter plants such as yellow gentian (*Gentiana lutea L.—Gentianaceae*), common centaury (*Erythraea centaurium L.—Gentianaceae*), buckbean (*Menyanthes trifoliata L.—Gentianaceae*), holy thistle (*Cnicus benedictus L.—Asteraceae*), chicory

(*Cichorium intybus L.–Asteraceae*), white horehound (*Marrubium vulgare L.–Lamiaceae*), dandelion (*Taraxacum officinale Web.–Asteraceae*), and common stinging nettle (*Urtica dioica L.–Urticaceae*). All these plants are nonpoisonous and are good for loss of appetite, emaciation, and poor digestion. They increase the flow of saliva and of the gastric juices, help the stomach to empty more slowly, and improve the efficiency of assimilation. As a result, the whole organism is strengthened.

But we must also mention the many poisonous bitter plants containing powerful alkaloids. Such alkaloids are very varied in their effects, and each one has a specific pharmacological (or *Prabhava*) action. Usually the action concerns a given organ or tissue or a certain disease. Examples of plants in this group are tobacco (*Nicotiana tabacum L.–Solanaceae*), deadly nightshade (*Atropa belladonna L.–Solanaceae*), opium poppy (*Papaver somniferum L.–Papaveraceae*) and woody nightshade (*Solanum dulcamara L.–Solanaceae*), to name but a few. Their use has to be left to qualified medical practitioners with sufficient knowledge and experience to prescribe the exact dose.

The same is true of plants producing bitter-tasting glycosides. The best known representatives of this group are foxglove (*Digitalis Spec.–Scrophulariaceae*), lily of the valley (*Convallaria majalis L.–Liliaceae*), and the common oleander (*Nerium oleander L.–Apocynaceae*), all of which contain principles that act on the heart.

Not always particularly bitter in taste, but definitely aligned with the stronger bitters by their action, are the saponin glycosides, which are blood purifying and expectorant and are promoters of resorption. Examples of plants in this group are soapwort (*Saponaria officinalis L.–Caryophyllaceae*), cowslip (*Primula veris L.–Primulaceae*), cyclamen (*Cyclamen europaeum L.–Primulaceae*), and horse chestnut (*Aesculus hippocastanum L.–Hippocastanaceae*).

I wish to reiterate the warning that great caution should be exercised with bitter herbs, and one needs to be very knowledgeable before venturing to employ any of them; because their *Prabhava* effect is stronger than all their other effects.

Most Indians reject toothbrushes and toothpaste in favor of *Nimba* (*Azadirachta indica Juss.–Meliaceae*), a large evergreen with pinnate leaves commonly found throughout India. Its twigs are sold daily in the markets. If we compare the typical gleaming smile and healthy teeth of the average Indian with those of his European counterpart, we may be forced to admit that dental hygiene with *Nimba* twigs is much to be preferred to our own method. The bark of the tree is a remedy for fevers and skin diseases, its fruits are good for hemorrhoids and ulcers, and its leaves are used for disinfecting and healing wounds. A great favorite is the powder known as *Pancha Nimba* (the five *Nimbas*), prepared from the root, bark, leaves, flowers, and fruit of the *Nimba* tree. These are pulverized, mixed in equal proportions, and made up into pills for *Pitta* diseases.

One of the most notable roots belonging to the 'bitter plants' is turmeric, or *Haridra* (*Curcuma longa L.—Zingiberaceae*). Turmeric is a very important ingredient in curry. In India any flavoring added as a sauce to vegetables or rice is called curry. Indian culinary art produces hundreds of such mixtures; they usually contain six or more spices of which *Haridra* is always one. Each morning in practically every Indian kitchen, a fresh curry is ground in the traditional manner by using a stone roller and a stone slab. Curry as known in Europe is a standardized, not too pungent mixture introduced by the English. The sturdy plant appears to have only a short stem because its main portion runs under the soil as a rhizome. Its root is thick, yellow, and tuberous and has many fingerlike projections. The yellow coloring matter is contained in the short, fleshy tubers. The simple leaves grow in tufts; their expanded petioles form a sheath around the stem. The flowers have pink bracts. The basic flavor of *Haridra* is bitter, but it is also pungent and astringent. Its properties are light, dry, and keen; medicinally it is warming, and its product of digestion is pungent.

Turmeric is a good stomachic and regulates the appetite. As with ginger, small pieces of it can be chewed before meals. When powdered and stirred into hot milk, *Haridra* helps sore throats and allays the symptoms of colds, coughs, and chills in general. In the diet of diabetics, too, turmeric has a very positive effect. It is used both internally and externally in rheumatism. *Haridra* also has antiallergencic properties. In nettle rash and eczema, a paste made from yoghurt and *Haridra* has proved very effective when smeared on the skin. This remarkable plant has a further property: it staunches the bleeding from cuts very quickly. Finally, *Haridra* also enters into a traditional cosmetic preparation when pulverized and mixed with coriander powder and sandalwood oil. If this preparation is massaged into the body after a hot bath, the skin shines.

Coriander (*Coriandrum sativum L.—Apiaceae*) is another familiar ingredient of curry powders. This very old spice, mentioned in ancient Egyptian and Hebrew writings, presumably originated in the Mediterranean region. Coriander is an aromatic herb growing about three feet high. The tiny white or purple flowers cluster in secondary umbels. Under slight pressure the round fruit splits into two hemispheres. It is the fruit that is used in medicine.

The taste of the coriander fruit is bitter, a little pungent, sweet, and faintly astringent. Its therapeutic action is not hot but is cooling; the digestive product is sweet. It is a diuretic, carminative (curing flatulence), and appetizer. A decoction of coriander fruit is dispensed in fevers for the burning sensation in the body. The decoction is also used as an eyewash in conjunctivitis. Coriander powder stems hemorrhoidal bleeding.

Jatamansi (*Nardostachys jatamansi DC.–Valerianaceae*) is also known as Indian spikenard. This herb, which attains a height of two feet, is indigenous to Himalayan slopes and valleys at heights of up to 13,000 feet. The part used is the woody rhizome, which is brown and pilose (hairy) and exhales a very charactistic odor. Its taste is bitter, astringent, and sweet; its properties are light, keen, and viscous. The therapeutic action is cooling, and the product of digestion is pungent. *Jatamansi* is an antispasmodic and tonic, and is therefore prescribed in nervous cramps, as well as to regulate digestion, micturition, and the menstrual flow. *Jatamansi* is also an ingredient in some of our teas.

Kutaja (*Holarrhena antidysenterica Wall.–Apocynaceae*) is a small tree growing at heights of 4,000 feet. It is often used in reforestation because of its hardiness. One characteristic of *Kutaja* is that any part of the tree will exude a white, milky juice when injured. The bark and seeds are used in medicine. The bark, which is sold under the name *Kurchi* in Indian markets, is a good remedy for diarrhea; the seeds are a febrifuge.

Kutaki or *Katuka* (*Picrorhiza kurroa Royle et Benth.–Scrophulariaceae*) are names of a small herb growing widespread in the Himalayas from Kashmir to Sikkim at heights of up to 13,000 feet. Only the rhizome is used therapeutically. When cut it characteristically exhibits a light center surrounded by dark, light, and dark rings successively. The rhizome is a tonic for the liver and gall bladder and helps in jaundice—provided the patient is free of fever. It is a mild aperient and stimulates the appetite.

The leaves of the evergreen shrub, *Vasa* (*Adhatoda vasica Ness.–Acanthaceae*), are incorporated in herbal teas used for treating coughs. They are expectorant and antispasmodic. *Vasa* has also won a place in the homeopathic repertory.

Kantakari (*Solanum xanthocarpium L.–Solanaceae*) is another ingredient of cough medicines. Like the potato and tomato, it is a member of the nightshade family. Its indications are cough, asthma, chest pain, and fever.

Yet another of the nightshades is *Brihati* (*Solanum indicum L.*), a yellow-fruited bush the root of which is employed as an expectorant in cough mixtures. *Brihati* is a component of the famed ten-root mixture *Dasa mula* which, since its leading taste is astringent, will be left to the next chapter for discussion.

A very effective bitter tonic is the poisonous Indian aconite, *Vatsanabha* (*Aconitum ferox Wall.—Ranunculaceae*). It is used after its roots have been pretreated by steeping them in cow's milk to draw out the poison.

The nonpoisonous aconite *Ativisa* (*Aconitum heterophyllum Wall.—Ranunculaceae*) is prescribed for children suffering from diarrhea accompanied by fever and is also used as a stomachic. Unlike the rhizome of *Vatsanabha*, its rhizome makes the tongue tingle.

Saptaparna (*Alstonia scholaris R. Br.—Apocynaceae*) is an evergreen tree growing eighty feet high which thrives in a wet climate. It contains a bitter milky juice. Its bark is used as a bitter in diarrhea and malarial fever and is also helpful in snakebite. A paste made of the bark of the *Saptaparna* tree is often applied to abscesses.

The roots of the climber, *Kebuka* (*Costus speciosus* [*Koen.*] *Sm.—Scitaminaceae*), tonicize, promote digestion, expel worms, and stimulate the uterus.

The well-known jasmine, *Jati* (*Jasminum grandiflorum L.—Oleaceae*) is one of the bitter herbs. The juice of the fresh leaves and flowers is worked into a disinfectant ointment which promotes the healing of wounds.

At least as well-loved as the sweet scent of jasmine is the aroma exhaled by the roots of the *Khaskhas* grass, *Usira* (*Vetivera zizanoides L.—Gramineae*). During the hot season, the *Usira* roots are placed in the window and are sprinkled with water so that the room may be filled with a refreshing fragrance. When the oil from this root is taken internally, it is useful in *Pitta* diseases. Externally, a paste made from powdered *Usira* roots and water is employed as a cooling application in fevers; it also has a reputation as a cosmetic.

In India lykodermia, a pigment disorder of the skin, is a common and much feared complaint. White patches occur which often cover entire parts of the body and are especially upsetting when they involve the face. One remedy is the bitter plant, *Bakuchi* (*Psoralea corylifolia L.—Leguminosae*), a small herb with black kidney-shaped fruit that is used both externally and internally.

Arka (*Calotropis gigantea—Asclepediaceae*) is a widely disseminated shrub with white to grey-violet flowers. The therapeutic property of

Arka is heating; therefore, it calms *Kapha*-linked *Pitta* disorders and does not foment *Vata*. The leaves and roots of this shrub supply remedies for coughs and asthma and are prescribed like digitalis for heart trouble.

Sandalwood oil occurs naturally only in South India; therefore in North India and in the Himalayan states the essential oil of *Aguru* (*Aquilaria agallocha Roxb.—Thymeliaceae*) is used as a substitute. This is carminative and astringent and is given for diarrhea and as a tonic.

Many of the major bitter herbs are also well-known in Europe. Thus, the active principles isolated from rauwolfia and from nux vomica have become indispensable items in our pharmacopoeia. Both plants have, of course, long been known in India for their medicinal virtues.

Charaka himself mentioned the 'Indian snakeroot', *Sarpagandha* (*Rauwolfia serpentina L.—Apocynaceae*). The action of rauwolfia is predominantly *Prabhavic*. The small bush with red berries grows best around the foot of the Himalayas. The roots are gathered from three-year-old shrubs. Their effect is tranquilizing and hypotensive (lowering blood pressure). Rauwolfia root is frequently combined with calamus root as a cure for snakebite and insect stings and also for diarrhea and fever.

Kupilu (*Strychnos nux vomica L.—Loganiaceae*) comes from a big tree with orange-colored fruit and with seeds resembling hairy white buttons. These seeds are the 'poison nuts;' they are very toxic and traditionally undergo a complicated pre-treatment before use. First of all they are boiled for seven days—not in water but in cow's urine. Next they are thoroughly washed, the seed coats are taken away, and the seeds are halved so that the cotyledons can be removed. The seeds are then ground to a powder, which is roasted in ghee until brown. The dosage is from thirty to one hundred milligrams in *Vata* diseases such as paralysis and joint pains, and (even) impaired hearing. *Kupilu* stimulates the muscles and sharpens all the senses.

The dried leaf juice of the aloe (*Aloe barbadensis Mill.—Liliaceae*) is sold in our pharmacies as an aperient. The plant's Sanskrit name, *Kuari* means 'maiden.' Its main taste is bitter, and its subsidiary taste is sweet; its properties are heavy, oily, and sticky. In India the whole plant is used. Small doses are employed as a stomachic and tonic; large doses as a laxative, and, indirectly, as a vermifuge. The fresh leaf juice is cooling; the fresh leaves themselves are a domestic remedy for childhood liver disorders.

'Indian' valerian, *Tagara* (*Valeriana wallichi DC.—Valerianaceae*), grows up to two meters high. Its thick, hairy root is sold on the Indian market under the name of *Sugandha Bala*, or 'sweet-smelling maiden.' The main taste is bitter, and subsidiary tastes are pungent, sweet, and astringent. Its properties are light, oily, and mobile. Therapeutically, it is heating, and its digestive product is pungent. The root, like that of its European cousin, is used as an anticonvulsive sedative and is therefore used in disorders triggered by an excess of *Vata*.

Tuvaraka (*Hydnocarpus wightiana Blume*—Flacourtiaceae) is a herb which is especially significant for the so-called developing countries because the oil from its seeds is an effective treatment for leprosy. It is applied externally and is also given as an injection. Interestingly enough, both forms of treatment are mentioned in the classical Ayurvedic writings of Susruta—evidence that injections were known and used in ancient India.

The term *Medhya Rasayan* is applied to plants that are now called psychedelic or 'mind-expanding.' In bygone times the effects of such plants were thought to be magical; they are the miraculous herbs of old tales and legends. There are four particularly noteworthy members of the *Medhya Rasayan* group which have a bitter taste, with perhaps a touch of astringency. Their properties are light, oily, and mobile (exceptions to this rule will be mentioned where appropriate); therapeutically they are cold, and the product of digestion is sweet.

Brahmi (*Bacopa monieri L.*—Scrophulariaceae), a small herb growing only in very damp places, is known as '*Brahmi* of Bengal.' Like other drugs of this type, it is employed in epilepsy and as a calmative. However, another plant (*Centella asiatica*—Umbelliferae) is also called *Brahmi*, although the popular name is *Mandukarpani*, meaning 'froglike.' The reason for the latter name is the way the plant propagates itself: its roots take a curving leap out of the ground, so to speak, and return to earth only to jump out again in the same fashion. *Mandukarpani* is dispensed chiefly in nervous disorders, but is also used for skin complaints and diarrhea.

The third *Medhya Rasayan* plant is a native of Europe, too—the sweet flag, also known as 'German ginger.' Growing in marshy places, *Vacha* (*Acorus calamus L.*—Araceae) was mentioned by Charaka and was also celebrated in Old Persian songs. We also find it discussed in the famous herbal of the Chinese Emperor Shen Nung, who lived three thousand seven hundred years before the birth of Christ. The plant has a perennial creeping rhizome which grows in the wet mud flanking lakes and rivers. From the end of the rhizome sprout numerous sword-shaped leaves, which attain a height of some three feet. The three- or four-noded stem bears in its center a yellow-green spadix about two to three inches long.

The fruits are red berries, but these seldom ripen in Central European conditions. Very early in spring, before the leaves have developed, or in late autumn, the rhizomes are 'harvested' by being hooked out of the mire. The root is trimmed and cleaned of its excrescences and is then chopped into finger-length sections and dried. The surface of the root is brownish green, but inside it is white, soft, and spongy. The taste is bitter; however, it is much milder when dried.

First and foremost, *Vacha* is a stomachic and is good for the treatment of gastritis, enteritis, chronic dyspepsia, loss of appetite or an aversion to food even when hunger is felt, for signs of gastric fermentation, and for relaxed stomach muscles. At the same time, the excretion of urine is promoted, bile secretion and the flow of bile are normalized, and pockets of gas are dispersed. The natural consequences of all these benefits are the correction of a disturbed metabolism, the stimulation of blood circulation, and an essential improvement of anemia.

Sweet flag rhizome is often added to baths to soothe 'jangled nerves' or, more specifically, to relieve nervous insomnia, neurasthenia, and painful periods. In folk medicine, the infusion is credited with great powers of strengthening the memory.

Ayurveda reports the taste of *Vacha* as bitter and pungent, its properties as light, keen, and mobile, its therapeutic action as hot, and its digestive product as pungent. In its effects on the *Tri Doshas*, sweet flag is calming on *Vata* and *Kapha* (even though the bitter taste usually intensifies *Vata*), and it reduces *Pitta* by excretion. The powdered rhizome and the fresh leaves are used medicinally as cordial bitters and are carminative and antispasmodic; their strengthening (*Medhya Rasayan*) action extends from improvement of the cerebral function to expansion of consciousness and the allaying of nervous irritation.

Shankhapuspi (*Convolvulus pluricaulis* Choisy—*Convulvulaceae*) is also *Medhya Rasayan*. *Shankha* means 'mussel shell' and *Puspi* means 'bloom.' The whole plant is used. It strenghens the cerebral function, is mind expanding, and is a favorite prescription for epilepsy, hysteria, and insomnia.

Many Indian gardens are graced by the presence of *Paribhadraka* (*Erythrina indica* Lam.—*Leguminoseae*), the coral tree. Growing to a height of up to sixty feet, it has branches which, although almost leafless from January to March, brighten the early months with a splash of coral-red blossom and are alive with twittering birds. The leaves and bark are the parts used. The principle taste is bitter, the subsidiary taste pungent; the property is light, the therapeutic action hot, and the product of digestion pungent. *Paribhadraka* enjoys a reputation as an antidote to strychnine. Its leaves are aperient; they also encourage the start of menstruation and of milk secretion. The bark is helpful in gallstone colic and liverishness, and is an expectorant, febrifuge, and vermifuge.

23

ASTRINGENCY

The Taste Kasaya, with Examples of Its Action

The astringent taste, *kasaya*, arises from the elements air and earth and possesses the basic energies of light, cold, and dry. Astringency causes a stiffening and contraction of the tongue and throat, a dry mouth, a feeling of heaviness, and diminished secretion of saliva. It is maintained in the Ayurvedic classics that astringency produces clarity. An excess of the astringent taste can lead to pains in the region of the heart. Its chemical vehicles are the tannins.

In acting on the *Tri Doshas*, astringency reinforces *Vata* through its element air and its light energy but reduces *Pitta* through its cold energy and *Kapha* through its dry energy. In its effect on the body tissues it is catabolic and resorbent, especially where the components of fatty tissue, muscle fat, and bone marrow are concerned.

Generally speaking, astringent-tasting things are healing and aid the whole healing process; they are absorptive, diminish the amount of urine, and normalize skin pigmentation. Astringent remedies are given for diarrhea and dysentery, hemorrhages and wounds, a pathological increase of the flow of urine, and breathing disorders. Contraindications are disturbed *Vata*, loss of appetite, and general debility.

Immoderate use of astringent items can give rise to several disorders: cardiac pain, dry mouth, hoarse voice, constipation, impotence, loss of oxygen saturation of the blood, flatulence, spermatemphraxis (an impediment to the discharge of semen), retention of urine and feces, debility, decay, ankylosis (stiffness of joint surfaces impairing movement), paralysis, and lowness of spirits.

Medicinal plants containing tannin are used by us chiefly in inflammations of exposed mucous membranes and in wounds, burns, skin diseases, excessive perspiration, diarrhea, and dysentery. Tannins astringe or 'tan' the superficial cell layers and thus reduce the irritability of the cells and make them more resistant. The glandular secretions cease and a dryness is produced; there is also a local anaesthetic effect due to reduced functioning of the sensitive nerve endings.

In the oral cavity, tannins make the tissues feel tight and reduce the sense of taste. They have an antiseptic action for inflammatory conditions or, to be more precise, they inhibit or neutralize putrefaction. In wounds germs are prevented from penetrating to the deeper layers. In diarrhea, decomposition in the intestines is inhibited, and the mucous membrane there is made more tough and leathery. Toxic materials are kept at bay, and peristalsis is reduced.

Among the most important astringents used medically by Europeans is the bark of two species of oak (*Quercus robur L.—Fagaceae* and *Quercus petreae L.—Fagaceae*). A decoction of the bark from young twigs is employed in poultices and baths and is taken internally as a tisane.

In tormentil (*Potentilla erecta L.—Rosaceae*) we have another example from Europe. The knotty root is the part of the yellow-flowered herb used. A blood-red stain appears when the root is freshly cut or broken. The plant is a valuable remedy in bowel infections, jaundice, liver swellings, and inflammations of the mucous membranes. It is also prescribed as a blood purifier in rheumatism, gout, and diabetes.

Dried bilberries or whortleberries (*Vaccinium myrtillus L.—Ericaceae*) are very rich in tannin and are given for diarrhea. Their advantage is that, because of the slow release of this tannin—which does not take place until the intestines are reached—they place no strain on the stomach.

Not only are the leaves of the wild strawberry (*Fragaria vesca L.—Rosaceae*) and of the raspberry (*Rubus ideaus L.—Rosaceae*) and blackberry (*Rubus fructicosus L.—Rosaceae*) used as substitutes for Chinese green tea, but they are prized for their astringent and diuretic action.

The houseleek (*Sempervivum tectorum*) forms an astringent remedy for wounds and inflammations when the freshly bruised leaves are applied. It owes its common name to its reputation as a lightning conductor: in bygone times its main function was to prevent the roofs of houses from being struck in thunderstorms. More than a superstition? Yes, the point discharge from the tops of its clustered leaves would have helped to equalize the local atmosphere tension.

The nuts of the walnut tree (*Juglans regia L.—Juglandaceae*) are sweet; they are an important spare diet with a high content of protein, carbohydrates, mineral salts, and vitamins. The astringent parts are the leaves of the tree and the green rinds of the walnuts, which are used medicinally both internally and externally.*

Other astringent plants are sage (*Salvia officinalis L.—Lamiaceae*) and

---

* Translator's note: In obstinate skin complaints, diarrhea, sore throat etc.

St. John's wort (*Hypericum perforatum L.–Hypericaceae*), the astringency of which assists the action of their essential oils. Sage tea regulates the perspiration,* reduces lactation, and also makes an excellent gargle. A decoction of St. John's wort is antiseptic, diuretic, and calmative. Hypericum oil is used externally to heal wounds and help scar formation.

If astringent Asiatic plants were entered in a beauty contest, first prize would surely be won by the cotton tree *Shalmali* (*Bombax malabaricum DC.–Bombacaceae*) from the Malabar coast. For much of the year this tall, thorny tree is leafless. In January it produces big red blooms with five irregularly shaped petals. Each flower has about sixty anthers. The fingerlike fruits appear in April and turn from green to brown. They supply the 'Indian kapok' which is used for stuffing cushions. Because of their astringency the roots and bark of the *Shalmali* tree are used for diarrhea and dysentery, and are also used as a tonic. A paste is applied externally to remove skin impurities.

Another wonderfully fine plant is *Dhataki* (*Woodfordia fructicosa Kurz.–Lythraceae*), a bush with copper-red flowers that look like flames. These flowers are employed as astringents and are also used for dyeing.

Astringency is a property of the many species of Indian fig, of which *Udumbara* (*Ficus racemosa L.–Moraceae*) is the most significant from a medical point of view. The bark of this tree is given for cattle plague, its roots help in diarrhea, and its fruits regulate the stomach and cure flatulence.

Vata (*Ficus bengaliensis L.–Moraceae*) is the old Sanskrit name of the banyan tree which, as we shall see, is with good reason also called the 'strangler fig.' This native of South and West India, with large, pale-veined leathery leaves, might seem to the superficial observer to have no flowers but only fruit in the shape of small figs—the latter being very attractive to most species of birds. Sometimes bird dung containing the seeds will fall on some other tree, which then plays host to the banyan. However, the latter is no ordinary parasite: initially, the host is not harmed by the insignificant seedling. But it soon develops long thready roots which, although at first waving innocently in the breeze, start forming a net that becomes denser and denser and quickly attains vast dimensions once the aerial roots have reached the ground and the *Ficus* plant is fully self-supporting and no longer needs to draw nourishment from its host. Now the drama reaches its climax. The

---

* Translator's note: Mrs C. D. Leye, *Green Medicine* (Faber & Faber, 1952), says that 'Sage is an excellent remedy for . . . the shaking fits of ague and the night sweats of tubercular subjects'.

mighty banyan squeezes the host tree with titanic strength and incorporates it in itself.* The strangler fig greatly extends the territory once occupied by its victim and is highly valued as a source of shade; so much so, in fact, that in India the word banyan has become a synonym for 'market' because markets are often held under its cover.

An important species of fig in India is *Asvattha* (*Ficus religiosa*), the 'sacred fig tree.' It has long-petioled leaves which hang fluttering in the wind like tiny fans. It is planted for religious reasons in India and Sri Lanka. The Indians associate the *Asvattha* with Brahma, Vishnu, and Shiva (Vishnu is said to have been born under such a fig tree). The Buddhists call it a Bo tree and relate that while sitting beneath its shade one day in the sixth century BC, a certain Prince Siddhartha found the enlightenment that won him the title Gautama Buddha.

Arjuna (*Terminalia arjuna—Combretacea*) is another sacred tree, and it may not be felled. Only the bark is used medicinally. This is white on the outside and reddish on the inside. As a decoction made with milk and water, it is used for hemorrhages and is an excellent heart tonic (its *Prabhava* effect). *Arjuna*, after whom it was named, was the noblest and bravest warrior in the national epic the *Mahabharata*, and shares his characteristics with the tree: his courage has its counterpart in the heart-strengthening properties of the latter.

The bark of siris or *Shirisa* (*Albizzia lebbek L.—Mimosaceae*) is highly valued as a remedy, too. *Charaka* himself reported it as a good antidote for poisonings, snake bite, scorpion stings, and insect bites and said that it was an outstanding treatment for bronchial asthma and skin complaints such as eczema.† Modern practice confirms this old knowledge.

Distributed throughout India is the catechu tree, *Babula* (*Acacia catechu Wild.—Mimosaceae*), which grows to a height of forty feet. Its gummy juice is the Indian equivalent of the gum arabic obtained from the African species *Acacia senegal*. The *Babula* tree is equipped to defend itself both against extreme drought and grazing cattle. Its feathery leaves can close so as to reduce transpiration very considerably during periods of great heat; and at browsing level its lower branches are well armed with daunting thorns. The typical globular flowers (known to us a

---

* Translator's note: 'In very old specimens the leaves and head of the palmyra are seen emerging from the trunk of the banyan tree, as if they grew from it. These the Hindus regard with reverence and call them holy marriages.' (Major H. Drury, *The Useful Plants of India*, Madras, 1858).

† Translator's note: In other words, it contains an antihistamine.

mimosa in other species of acacia) appear from June to November. The ripe legumes contain up to a dozen seeds. The bipinnate leaves have stipulary thorns. When the bark is cut, a sticky juice flows out, and this 'gum' is employed in *Kapha* and *Pitta* disorders; it is styptic and astringent and makes a good tonic. It may be used both externally and internally, externally as a paint or gargle and internally for disordered stomachs and diarrhea.

The resinous gum exuded by the incense tree *Sallaki (Boswellia serrata Roxb.—Burseraceae)* is also an astringent remedy used for skin diseases, rheumatism, and nervous complaints. Until frankincense was replaced by Peruvian balsam in the sixteenth century, that and myrrh were among the most costly substances transported from continent to continent along the old caravan routes. The 'wise men from the east' of the New Testament carried this treasure to Bethlehem. And the gum of myrrh or *Guggulu (Commiphora mukul Hook.—Burseraceae)* which they also brought—a strong-smelling gum obtained by cutting the tree's scaly grey branches—is used therapeutically, too. Its principle taste is astringent, its by-taste bitter, and its special field of application is all rheumatic disorders.

A most frequently used remedy is a blend of three fruits: *Tri Phala*. One of the ingredients, *Amalaki (Emblica officinalis Gaertn.—Euphorbiaceae)* has already been described in the chapter on *amla*, the sour taste. The other two fruits in the *Tri Phala* mixture are *kasaya* (astringent), and each has a specific action.

Bibhitaki (Terminalia belerica Gaertn.—Combretaceae) are the brown fruits of a tall tree, which have a sweet effect after digestion and therefore do not excite *Pitta*. They are employed in *Kapha* diseases, especially in certain cases of ophthalmia.

The third fruit in the *Tri Phala* is *Haritaki (Terminalia chebula Retz.—Combretaceae)*. The yellow-green fruits come from a medium-sized tree and exhibit five very characteristic furrows. The fruits are used without their seeds, as are the *Bihitaki* fruits just mentioned. The principle taste is astringent and is accompanied by the tastes bitter, pungent, sweet, and sour. Like the two other *Tri Phala* fruits, its product of digestion is sweet, and all three help in disorders of all three *Doshas*. On its own, *Haritaki* acts as a mild laxative and is good for problems with the eyes, hair loss, chronic fever, and chronic diarrhea. It is also recommended as an antidote for the troubles attendant on old age and can be used throughout the year if a second item is combined with it according to the season: in winter, ginger; in early spring, pepper; in spring, honey; in autumn, refined sugar.

Tri Phala, the powdered mixture of the dried fruits of the three species mentioned above, is used mainly in *Kapha* and *Pitta* disorders. It is very beneficial for diseases of the kidneys and bladder, diabetes, skin diseases, eye complaints, intermittent fevers, loss of appetite, constipation, and dysentery; it also improves iron resorption.

An equally popular mixture is *Dasa mula*, the ten roots. We have already taken a look at some of the roots concerned in the chapters on the tastes sweet and pungent—these are roots of grasses and form the set known as the 'five small roots.' The 'five great roots' of the *Dasa mula* are tree roots of which the cortices are used in equal parts as a freshly made decoction or as a fermented preparation for keeping. In taste they are astringent, bitter, and sweet; their properties are hot and light, and they reduce *Kapha* and *Vata*. These *Dasa mula* components are also extremely effective when used as simples. *Bilva* (*Aegle marmelos L.—Rutaceae*) is a thorny tree the leaves of which possess oil glands and exhale a pleasant scent. Its fruits are known as Bela fruit or 'Indian quinces.'

Its root cortex is calming and febrifuge. *Agni mantha* (*Premna integrifolica Roxb.—Verbenaceae*) has a root the cortex of which is celebrated for its antiinflammatory and digestive properties. *Syonaka* (*Droxylum indicum—Bignoniaceae*) is a tree made conspicuous by its large sword-shaped fruit. Used on its own, the root cortex is prescribed in *Vata* diseases: as a bitter tonic in diarrhea and dysentery. The tall *Patala* tree (*Stereospermum suaveolens—Bignoniaceae*) has remarkably rough leaves. Its heavily scented flowers are used to make perfumed water. The root cortex is employed in *Vata* and *Kapha* disorders, but is used chiefly in the *Dasa Mula* mixture. The *Gamhara* tree (*Gmelina arborea—Verbenaceae*) has bittersweet fruits which are cooling and are used as a remedy for shortness of breath. The root cortex, the fifth component of the 'five great roots,' helps to cure fevers and indigestion.*

Madhu, or honey, is not only an important remedy in its own right, it is also a useful vehicle for other medications. The name *Madhu* identifies it with *madhura*, sweetness; as 'sweet as honey' we say. In actual fact, the taste of honey is a combination of both sweet and astringent, and, because of its effects, Ayurveda treats it as one of the astringent substances. Honey is energy giving and is stimulating to the digestion; it is cooling. It reduces *Kapha* and with it obesity. It cleans and heals

---

* Translator's note: '*Gmelina arborea* (*Roxb.*) . . . The root in decoction is used in fevers accompanying gouts or pains in the limbs. The powdered bark of the root is applied externally in gout.' (Major Heber Drury, *The Useful Plants of India*, Madras, 1858).

festering sores and assists the mending of fractured bones; it strengthens both the sight and the voice, acts as a heart tonic, and cures nausea, hiccups, poisoning, asthma, bronchitis, swellings, diarrhea and sleepiness.

Since it is made from nectar taken from many flowers, it may be regarded as a blend of the most varied healing substances. The classical texts distinguish eight different types of honey, each with their own special properties, according to the terrain, the patch of flowers, and the time of year in which the bees were gathering the nectar. We ourselves, of course, know various sorts of honey. The Ayurveda classics issue this warning: honey and milk should never be mixed with salt.

24

THE HEALER WITHIN

Ayurvedic Treatment Starts with the Healthy

Naturally, the exponents of every system of medicine would prefer to stop people from becoming ill. In rural China, for example, the doctor who is most respected is the one who has least to do, because the patients on his list remain hale and hearty.

Medical experts in industrialized countries have accomplished much in the field of preventive medicine during the last two centuries—we need think only of the fundamental improvement in hygiene and of the various types of inoculations to remind us of this. Unfortunately, however, the very developments making these triumphs possible have created conditions responsible for a host of new menaces to health, quite apart from having a hand in the so-called diseases of civilization.

In the classical Ayurvedic texts there are descriptions not only of the causes and treatment of diseases but also of many prophylactic measures. They lay down comprehensive rules for daily living: how to build 'healthy houses,' how to look after the well-being of livestock and crops, diet sheets, advice on the whole mode of life, and proposals for physical and spiritual exercise—all aimed at self-development and 'life-balance.' The regular routine of a 'classically' healthy day looks something like this:

- Rising before dawn (six to eight hours of sleep is enough).
- Cleaning the teeth with powdered herbs mixed with oil and salt.
- Washing the mouth, eyes, and face with vegetable extracts.
- Oil in the nose and ears, oil massage for the body and head.
- Physical exercises suited to the individual's constitution and condition and to the time of year.
- Bath—cold in summer and warm in winter.
- Selection of the right clothing.
- Religious devotions according to one's faith.
- Meal.
- Work, study.

- Meal.
- A walk.
- Sexual activity.
- Sleep

Great attention is paid to the seasons in order to avoid congestion in any of the *Doshas* particularly active at a given time of year.

Natural bodily functions—not only urination and defecation but also coughing, sneezing, weeping, laughing, yawning, and so on—should not be suppressed. But emotions such as anger, jealousy, cruelty, and the like must be held strongly in check.

The physical exercises mentioned in the Ayurvedic schedule are the Yoga asanas. Yoga is not a division of Ayurveda but is a completely self-contained branch of knowledge. Its greatest significance lies in the fact that it is a road to self-development which stresses physical, spiritual, and mental health. The value to preventive medicine of this method of attaining all-round well-being is obvious.

The first systematic description of the method is to be found in the Yoga-Sutra (Yoga Aphorisms) of Patanjali,[39] which dates from about the time of Christ's birth. In these aphorisms we are presented with the eight steps of Yoga.*

1 *Yama*: Reliability in daily life. Right conduct towards others. Mutual consideration and respect.

2 *Niyama*: Discipline in physical culture, diet, and daily activities.

3 *Asana*: A series of postures designed to train consciousness and the responsiveness of the body. The asanas are especially important for maintaining health and for revealing incipient disease.

4 *Pranayama*: Refinement of the art of breathing.

5 *Pratyahara*: Stilling of the sensations and thoughts.

---

* Translator's note: A German translation of the sutras is mentioned in the bibliography. English renderings of varying degrees of literalness have been published under the auspices of the Theosophical Society, e.g., *The Yoga-Sutra by Patanjali* (translation with Introduction, Appendix and Notes based upon several authentic commentaries) (Manilal Nabhubhai Dvivedi, sometime Professor of Sanskrta, Samaladasa College, published by Tookaram Tatya for the Bombay Theosophical Fund, 1890), and *The Yoga Aphorisms of Patanjali* (An interpretation by William Q. Judge assisted by James Henderson Connelly) (Second Point Loma Edition published by the Theosophical Publishing Company, Point Loma, Ca, USA, 1914) (first edition published 1893). There is also *Aphorisms of Yoga* by Bhagwan Shree Patanjali translated into English from the original in Sanskrit with a commentary by Shree Purohit Swami and an Introduction by W.B. Yeats (Faber and Faber, London, 1938—paperback edition 1973). Yeats himself mentions the translation by James Horton Woods published by the Harvard Press.

6   *Dharana*: Concentration.
7   *Dhyana*: Meditation.*
8   *Samadhi*: Raptness.

Two different causes could be responsible for disease:

* Exogenous: when a *Dosha* is thrown out of equilibrium by some outside influence (e.g., injury).
* Endogenous: when a *Dosha* is stirred up and spreads from its proper place in the body to establish itself in some tissue, organ, or channel, bringing about in the latter a change that reveals itself in measurable symptoms.

Three factors are said to unbalance the *Tri Doshas*:

1   Overstimulation or understimulation of the sense organs.
2   Misuse of the mind and senses and neglect of the body.
3   The influence of times such as day and night or the seasons of the year; also the influence of the age of the individual concerned and similar factors.

Should some disease manifest itself, Ayurveda abandons for the time its role of guardian of health and becomes an active healing system.

Ayurveda distinguishes six stages in the course of an illness. Western industrialized medicine waits for stage four to arrive before starting treatment. The traditional Indian physican (and his patients expect no less) sets to work in stages one, two, and three; naturally, the adoption of early measures greatly increases the chances of recovery. In these first three stages of disease development, 'radical' therapy (*Samsodhana*) is still practicable, but once the fourth stage—which rapidly gives way to the fifth—is reached, the treatment becomes 'palliative' (*Samsamana*). The disease must then take its course. All that can be done is to alleviate it and to accelerate the healing process.

Sata Kriyakala is the name given to the 'six-rung ladder' of disease. The first 'rung' is *Sancaya*, the stage of accumulation. In this initial phase there is an accumulation of a single *Dosha* in 'its own place' or an accumulation of several *Doshas* each in their own locations. *Vata* increases in the rectum and colon. *Pitta* increases in the small intestine, pancreas, and liver. *Kapha* increases in the stomach. The factors responsible for the respective accumulations of the *Doshas* have the

---

*   Translator's note: John Mumford, *Psychosomatic Yoga*, Thorsons, 1962, explains the true meaning of Dhyana as 'Sustained Concentration.'

same properties as the *Doshas* concerned. For instance, heat strengthens *Pitta*, whereas cold strengthens *Kapha* and *Vata*.

Sancaya can be recognized by certain symptoms. An accumulation of *Vata* creates a sensation of fullness in the lower abdomen, inflates it, and disturbs peristalsis. An accumulation of *Pitta* creates a feeling of heat without a measurable rise in temperature and leads to loss of the natural healthy 'glow.' An accumulation of *Kapha* makes itself known by a feeling of heaviness in the limbs accompanied by weakness and lethargy.

The second 'rung' is *Prakopa*, the stage of excitation. Roughly translated *Prakopa* means 'exceptional aggravation.' There is irritation of one or more *Doshas* which were accumulated in the previous stage, *Sancaya*. The excited *Doshas* are still in their original places; there has been no spread as yet. Causes of the development of a disease from the first to the second stage are such factors as dietary deficiencies, physical exertion, the influences of season and climate, mild physiological disturbances like indigestion and psychic irritation.

Prakopa's special symptoms are easier to recognize than are those of the first stage. Excited *Vata* causes abdominal pain accompanied by gurgling sounds. Excited *Pitta* causes a burning sensation, hot flushes, heartburn and pronounced thirst. Excited *Kapha* reveals itself in nausea and loss of appetite.

The third 'rung in the ladder of disease' is *Prasara*, the stage of spreading. In this stage *Vata* is the dynamic or driving principle, and it is able to move the two other *Doshas* and diffuse them through the body. In total, thirteen modes of spreading are recognized, i.e., spreadings of each and all of the *Doshas* and of the blood in every possible combination. From this point of view, *Charaka* defines blood as the active vehicle, and *Susruta* counts it among the *Doshas* as a 'fourth force.'

Pronounced spreading shows certain symptoms. The spreading of *Vata* is seen in a swollen abdomen. The spreading of *Pitta* manifests itself in a feeling of heat and indigestion accompanied by a bad body odor. The spreading of *Kapha* is followed by digestive disorders and nausea and frequently by depression.

The fourth 'rung' is *Stana Samsraya*, the stage of localization. The fermented and diffused *Doshas* arrive at certain tissue structures and are retained in certain ducts or capillaries. A struggle ensues between the aggressive *Doshas* and the tissues that are congested by them. This is when the first clear symptoms of illness appear and the trouble can no longer be ignored. Our allopathic Western physicians call it the prodromal stage. The fourth 'rung' leads quickly to the fifth 'rung,' or

Vyakti, the stage of manifestation. The symptoms are then so salient that one is able to measure them qualitatively.

Finally we have *Bheda*, the stage of complications. It is here that the further course of the disease is decided. The possibilities are healing, complications, secondary disease, a chronic condition, or death.

There is no order of health corresponding to the development of disease. Health does not run any course; it is a labile condition, depending not only on the body but on the entire personality. We are coming to realize more and more clearly that a decisive dimension of health lies in ourselves and not in the drugstore. There is no way of achieving well-being of body and mind through intravenous injections, nor can the doctor write a prescription for holistic health. The latter is gained by making the best of life's ups and downs, by adopting a sensible regimen, by deliberately relaxing when stressed, by cultivating harmonious human relationships, and by finding life meaningful.

'The responsibility for getting well and staying well mainly belongs to the sufferer, to the patient, to the individual himself. We ought not to take it for granted so easily that health is something which can be purchased, or to blame our 'incompetent doctor' because he has failed in his 'duty' of restoring us to health.'[40]

External factors can do no more than help or hinder. The true healer is within us. This realization, which has always been inherent in Ayurveda, corresponds to the 'change in paradigms' which, according to Marilyn Ferguson, is occurring in many areas of knowledge: 'To put it plainly, a paradigm change is a new way of thinking about an old problem . . . A new paradigm embraces a principle which, although always present, had hitherto remained unrecognized. It contains the old as one aspect of itself, as a partial truth about how things function, while at the same time allowing that things can behave quite differently. With its broader perspective, the new paradigm transforms both the traditional knowledge and the awkward new observations, and thus removes their apparent contradictions.'[41]

The unconditional necessity for new ways of looking at and thinking about things is insisted on by Fritjof Capra, too: 'Humanity can survive only if it makes a fundamental change in its manner of life. This firstly demands a different way of thinking, a different 'perception' of the world. Namely, one that is complex instead of linear, in networks and curves instead of in the unidirectional straight lines and zigzags of statistics. Qualitative values must replace quantitative measurements. The world is more than the sum of its parts.'[42]

Now qualitative values are exceedingly important in Ayurveda, which means that becoming involved with this system of medicine will probably entail a paradigm change, or a change in our mental scheme of things—a necessary step for us to take today.

Ayurveda knows many simple, natural preventive measures for keeping the body in good trim. In the ideal case a person would lead a life that furthered his or her personal development and ensured pleasant social relationships.

According to Ayurveda, the roots of all diseases are activities which first, are not suited to the occasion (day, season, time of life); second, are not congenial; and third, involve inappropriate associations with sense objects.

Ayurveda also maintains that mental and physical health can be preserved sheerly by attentiveness: attentiveness to how we use the senses, adapt our daily routine to the demands of our environment, plan our diet, and respond to internal and external rhythms. Great stress is also laid on regular sleep and on bodily exercise (Yoga).

The object of Ayurveda is to assist nature. All the means used for cures do no more than support natural processes; they do not irritate nor do they substitute for or suppress what the body can do for itself.

The various forms of treatment in Ayurveda cover all conceivable possibilities including:

- *Ausadha*: treatment with medicinal plants and drugs.
- *Anna*: treatment by strict dieting.
- *Vihara*: various exercises.

Therapy (*Upasaya*) can be:

1 Opposed to the cause of the disease.
2 Opposed to the disease itself.
3 Opposed both to the cause and to the disease.
4 Similar to the cause of the disease.
5 Similar to the disease itself.
6 Similar both to the cause and to the disease.

All the principles of allopathy, homeopathy, and naturopathy are contained in these principles. The methods can be combined in forty-two ways.

One Ayurvedic saying runs like this: 'There is nothing within the range of thought and experience that cannot be used as a medicine or remedy.'[43] This recognizes that all existing phenomena have an influence on human makeup—physical, physiological, mental, and emotional. Love, hate, eating, drinking, drugs, fasting, massage, exercise, pleasant or unpleasant experiences or situations, social, climatic, or geographical conditions, positive or negative criticism, faith in God or the lack of it, neutral or evil thoughts—there is nothing that cannot be tried or used, that does not have a stronger or weaker influence on metabolism—there is nothing that cannot be employed in therapy.

Charaka writes on the importance of the ten questions. 'Why the ten questions? It is true that diseases are cured by medicines having properties opposed to the disease. However, this is not everything. It is important to make allowances for the site in which the medicinal plant grows, for the mental and physical condition of the patient, for the required dosage of the medicine, for the season of the year, and for the patient's age. If due consideration is not given to all these points, a medicinal plant cannot be relied upon to conquer the disease just because it possesses counteractive properties. This is why ten points bearing on the cure of the disease must be considered in every examination:

1 Which *Dosha* is out of balance?
2 Which medicinal herb is appropriate?
3 Place.
4 Time.
5 Capacity of resistance.
6 Physical constitution.
7 Diet.
8 Mental state.
9 Structure of the body.
10 Age.'

Ayurveda scorns the treatment of superficial symptoms and endeavours to bring about a radical cure by the pacification of an excessively excited *Dosha*. The destruction of disease germs is also not regarded as particularly sensible. The preferred aim of Ayurveda is to create conditions in which morbific agents can no longer multiply.

The healing processes of nature are supported in a threefold way. The first step is to excrete more waste matter more quickly. This is done by increasing *Kapha* through emetics which empty the stomach, by increasing *Pitta* through purgatives which clear the small intestine, or by increasing *Vata* through enemas which wash out the rectum and colon.

The second step is to calm the excited *Doshas* so that the disease processes cease. Increased *Kapha* is calmed by diets, medicinal plants, and therapies involving the tastes pungent, bitter, and astringent and the properties keen, hot, and dry. In increased *Pitta* the appropriate tastes are bitter, sweet, and astringent and the properties cold, mild, solid, and compact. For calming increased *Vata* we use the tastes salty, sour, and sweet and the properties hot, oily, heavy, compact, and slimy.

The third step consists of reinforcing the powers of resistance of mind and body so that the patient can overcome diseases and build up his or her resistance.

NOTES*

1 P. Lüth: *Das Medikamentenbuch.*
2 Article in *Die Zeit*, 26.2.1982.
3 Article in *Kurier*, 11.1.1981.
4 Ivan Illich: *Medical Nemesis.*
5 Rocque Lobo: *Yoga — Sensibilitätstraining für Erwachsene.*
6 Anthony Huxley: *Das phantastische Leben der Pflanzen.*
7 Jacques Attali: *Die kannibalische Ordnung.*
8 Marcel Bühler: *Geschäfte mit der Armut.*
9 *Der Spiegel*, No. 3, 1983.
10 Loc. cit.
11 *Bild der Wissenschaft*, September 1982.
12 *Entwicklungspolitische Nachrichten*, February 1983.
13 Six orthodox philosophical systems have sprung from the Upanishads: *Nyaya-Vaisesika* (originally two philosophical movements but later amalgamated), *Samkhya, Yoga, Purva Mimamsa, Uttara Mimamsa.*
14 Other names for *Purusha* are *Atman* and *Jiva.*
15 If *Sattwa*, or the principle of 'essence' dominates, qualities such as industry, reliability, erudition, realism, mildness, freedom of movement, and capacity for enthusiasm are displayed. If *Rajas*, the principle of 'energy' rules, and the person is restless and dissatisfied and tries to do more than one thing at a time; is undecided, selfish, irritable, insincere, and overemotional. A preponderance of *Tamas*, the principle of 'inertia', produces a despondent, phlegmatic person full of irregularities and laziness. These thumbnail sketches by Vagbhata are abstract formulae of pure character types that are never found in actuality, since all three principles iteract with one another in various proprotions.
16 *Manas* develops from *Sattwa Ahamkara* (the spirit ego) under the influence of *Rajas Ahamkara* (the energy ego). Between psyche and soul there is a strict distinction. Certainly the psyche is connected with the soul, but on the other hand it is a product of nutrition in the widest—thus also in the spiritual—sense.
17 Carmen Blacker and Michael Loewe: *Weltformeln der Frühzeit.*

* Further details are supplied in the bibliography.

[18] P.V. Sharma: *Introduction to Dravyaguna.*

[19] By 'principle (*Guna*) we chiefly understand one of the three fundamental properties of undifferentiated cosmic matter. *Sattwa, Rajas,* and *Tamas* are original properties of being which are always present. Only in a secondary sense does the word *Guna* stand for property in general. A table of the ten contrasting pairs can be found in Chapter 15.

[20] K.N. Udupa: 'Present Status of Research in Ayurveda', in Pandit Shiv Sharma: *Realms of Ayurveda.*

[21] Pandit Shiv Sharma: *Realms of Ayurveda.*

[22] Op. Cit.

[23] J. Rumpold: 'Die andere Heilkunst', alternative medicine. Austrian radio, 1982.

[24] Loc. Cit.

[25] Rocque Lobo: *Yoga—Sensibilitätstraining für Erwachsene.*

[26] *Prana:* the parasympathetic nerve plexus of the lungs.
Udana: the parasympathetic nerve plexus of the heart.
Samana: the parasympathetic nerve plexus of the sacral area.
Vyana: the motor nerves of the whole body.
(After K.D. Udupa: 'Der gegenwärtige Stand der Ayurveda-Forschung'—'The Current State of Ayurvedic Research').
[In the translator's opinion, this attempt to assimilate ancient concepts to modern anatomy and physiology is misguided becaused *prana, udana,* and the rest are forces, not nerve plexi, and it is impossible to understand them if we ignore their true definitions. *Samana,* for instance, is the northern gate to the heart, is known as 'on-breathing' (because it carries nutrients 'on' to their destination), and is located in the circle of the navel (through which nutrients are conveyed before birth) and stomach (through which nutrients are conveyed after birth). Thus it governs the digestion.]

[27] *Sadaka:* the catecholamines of the hypothalamus.
Alochaka: the sympathetic nerve plexus of the cerebral cortex.
Pachaka: the sympathetic nerve plexus of the colon.
Ranjaka: the sympathetic nerves of the liver and spleen.
Bhrajaka: the sympathetic nerve plexus of the skin.
(After K.N. Udupa: 'Der gegenwärtige Stand der Ayurveda-forschungs'—'The Current State of Ayurvedic Research'.)
[Once again, the modern interpretations do not seem to match the traditional descriptions, which tell us for example that 'Ranjaka . . . colours the rasa and turns it into blood', and '*Sadaka,* in the heart, causes sight, determination and memory'. (Dr. P. Kutumbiah, *Ancient Indian Medicine,* Orient Longmans Ltd., 1962). Western anatomy and physiology stops short at what can be physically observed and measured; Indian anatomy and physiology, on the other hand, seems to go beyond this; anyway, it is based in part on a different set of findings. Translator's note].

[28] *Kledaka:* regulates the secretions of the stomach and intestines.

Avalambaka: regulates the bronchial secretions.

Bodhaka: regulate the salivary and other secretions in the mouth.

Tarpaka: regulates fluid exchange in the brain.

Slesaka: operates in the spaces of the joints where synovial fluid is continually being produced and absorbed.

(After K. N. Udupa, op. cit.).

29 *Pancha* means 'five', and *Karma* here means 'action', hence 'the five actions'.

30 Rocque Lobo: *Yoga — Sensibilitätstraining für Erwachsene*.

31 After P.V. Sharma, *Introduction to Dravyaguna*.

32 Rocque Lobo, *Vorwort zu Ayurveda* by Ch. G. Thakkur.

33 Irving and Miriam Polster: *Gestalt Therapy Integrated*.

34 E. Kapfelsberger &. U. Pollmer: *Iss und stirb* (*Eat and Die*).

35 After P.V. Sharma: *Introduction to Dravyaguna*.

36 *Saumya*, the cold time of year, the 'wet season', is an Indian period of six months divided into *Varsa* (mid-July to mid-September), *Sharad* (mid-September to mid-November), and *Hemanta* (mid-November to Mid-January). During this period the earth gives off energy. *Saumya* is also a name given to the moon at this time: 'the moon with the cooling quality'.

37 *Agneya*, the hot time of year, is divided into *Shisira* (mid-January to mid-March), *Vasanta* (mid-March to mid-Mary), and *Grisma* (mid-May to mid-July). It is the time of drought and is ruled by the sun. During this period the earth absorbs energy.

38 The writings of Hippocrates (BC 460-377), the botanical studies of Theophrastus (BC 372-287), the works of Marcus Porcius Cato the Elder (BC 234-149) and of the natural philosopher Dioscorides (ca. AD 50), and the *Historia naturalis* of Pliny the Elder (AD 23-79).

39 Patanjali: *Die Wurzeln des Yoga, The Yoga-Sutra of Patanjali*, O.W. Barth, Bern—Munich 1979. [English-language editions are mentioned in *loc. cit.* All have valuable notes, those by Manilal Nathubhai Dvedi being particularly copious].

40 Gunter Emde: 'Kosmopathie', in Curare, Vol. 5, 1982.

41 Marilyn Ferguson: *Die sanfte Verschwörung*.

42 Fritjof Capra: *Wendezeit*.

43 Pandit Shiv Sharma: *Realms of Ayurveda*.

BIBLIOGRAPHY

Ansfelde, G.: Ayurvedisches Gewürzlexikon, Günther Koch, Braunschweig 1980.

Attali, Jacques.: Die kannibalische Ordnung, Campus, Frankfurt—New York 1981.

Ayurvedische Medizin, Die Grundprinzipien der, harrausgegeben vom Institut für Phänomenologie und Ganzheitswissenschaft, Stuttgart 1977.

Blacker, Carmen, und Loewe, Michael: Weltformeln der Frühzeit, Diederichs, Düsseldorf—Köln 1977.

Böhmig, Ulf: Das große Buch der natürlichen Heilkunde, Orace Pietsch, Wien 1981.

Braun, Hans.: Heilpflanzenlexikon für Ärzte und Apotheker, Gustave Fischer, Stuttgart—New York 1978.

Brooks, Charles, V. W.: Erleben durch die Sinne, Junfermann, Paderborn 1979.

Bühler, Marcel: Geschäfte mit der Armut, Medico International, Frankfurt 1983.

Caraka Samhita, (Agnivesas Caraka Samhita, Text with English translation & critical exposition based on Carakapani Datta's Ayurveda dipika), Chowkamba Sanskrit Series Office, Varanasi 1976.

Chaturvedi, G. N.: A Study of Panchakarma Therapy, Department of Kayachikitsa, Jamnagar 1959.

Dash, Bhagwan: Ayurvedic Treatment for Common Disease, Delhi Diary, New Delhi 1979.

Dash, Bhagwan: Fundamentals of Ayurvedic Medicine, Bansal & Co., New Delhi, 1978.

Dash, Bhagwan: Tibetan Medicine, Library of Tib. Works and Archives, Dharamsala 1976.

Derlon, Pierre: Die geheime Heilkunst der Zigeuner, Sphinx, Basel 1981.

Diepgen, P.: Geschichte der Medizin, Walter de Gruyter & Co., Berlin—Leipzig 1924.

Dönden, Yeshi: The Ambrosia Heart Tantra, Library of Tib. Works and Archives, Dharamsala 1977.

Ferguson, Marilyn: Die sanfte Verschwörung, Sphinx, Basel 1982.

Frauwallner, Erich: Geschichte der indischen Philosophie, Otto Müller, Salzburg 1953.

Geheimnisse und Heilkräfte der Pflanzen, Das Beste, Stuttgart 1978.

Gessner, O., und Orzechowski, G.: Gift- und Arzneipflanzen in Mitteleuropa, Carl Winter, Heidelberg 1974.

Gesundheit, Das Buch der ganzheitlichen, Scherz, Bern—Munchen—Wien 1982.

Goltz, Dietlinde: Versuch einer Grenzziehung zwischen Chemie und Alchemie, Franz Steiner, Wiesbaden 1968.

Grandjot, Werner: Reiseführer durch das Pflanzenreich der Tropen, Kurt Schroeder, Leichlingen b. Köln 1981.

Gupta, Shakti M.: Plant Myths, E. J. Brill, Leiden 1971.

Hakim, Mohammed Abdurrazzak: Principles and Practice of Traditional Systems of Medicine in India, WHO, Genf 1977.

Hoppe, H.A.: Drogenkunde, Walter de Gruyter, Berlin—New York 1975.

Huxley, Anthony: Das phantastische Leben der Pflanzen, dtv Sachbuch, München 1981.

Illich, Ivan: Medical Nemesis: The Expropriation of Health, Bantam, New York 1977.

Kapfelsperger, E., und Pollmer, U.: Iß und stirb, Chemie in unserer Nahrung, Kiepenheuer & Witsch, Köln 1982.

Kapfelsperger, E., und Pollmer, U.: Iß und stirb, Chemie in unserer Nahrung, Kiepenheuer & Witsch, Köln 1982.

Langbein, K./Martin, H. P./Weiss, H./Werner, R.: Gesunde Geschäfte, Die Praktiken der Pharmaindustrie, Kiepenheuer & Witsch 1981.

Lobo, Rocque: Yoga—Sensibilitätstraining für Erwachsene, Hueber-Holzemann, München 1978.

_____: Prana 1980, O. W. Barth/Scherz, Bern—München—Wien 1979.

_____: Prana 1981, O. W. Barth/Scherz, Bern—München—Wien 1980.

_____: Prana 1982/83, Du Mont, Köln 1982.

Lüth, P.: Das Medikamentenbuch, Rowohlt, Reinbek 1980.

Mahabharata, Indiens großes Epos, Diederichs, Düsseldorf—Köln 1978.

Manadhar, N.P.: Medicinal Plants of Nepal, Himalaywas, Ratnar Pustak Bhandar, Kathmandu 1980.

Medicinal Plants of India, Vol. 1, Indian Council of Medical Research New Delhi, New Delhi, 1976.

Mosig, A./Schramm, G.: Der Arzneipflanzen- und Drogenschatz Chinas und die Bedeutung des Pen- Ts'ao Kang-Mu, Volk und Gesundheit, Berlin 1955.

Müller, R. F. G.: Medizin der Inder in kritischer Übersicht, Indo-Asian Studies Part 2, International Academy of Indian Culture, New Delhi 1965.

Nanal, B. P.: Grundlagen des Ayurveda, Förderverein für Yoga und Ayurveda, München 1980.

Ohsawa, G.: Zen Makrobiotik, Franz Thiele, Hamburg 1976.

Patel, Bhulabhai: Mineralien und Chemikalien in der indischen Pharmazie, Pharmaziegeschichtliches Seminar der Technischen Hochschule Braunschweig, Braunschweig 1963.

Petersohn, L., und H.: Für eine andere Medizin, Fischer alternativ, Frankfurt 1981.

Polster, Irving and Miriam: Gestalt Therapy Integrated: Contours of Theory and Practice, Random, New York 1974.

Ray, P./Gupta, H. N./Roy, M.: Susruta Samhita, A Scientific Synopsis, Indian National Science Academy, New Delhi 1980.

Sharma, P. V.: Introduction to Dravyaguna, Chowkhamba orientalia, Varanasi 1976.

Sharma, Pandit Shiv: Realms of Ayurveda, Arnold Heinemann, New Delhi 1979.

Schneider, A.: Das grüne Geheimnis, München—Wien—Basel 1966.

Sigerist, Henry E.: Anfänge der Medizin, Europa, Zürich 1963.

Singh, T. B./Chunekar, K. C.: Glossary of Vegetable Drugs in Brhattrayi, Chowkhamba Sanskrit Series Office, Varanasi 1972.

Storl, Wolf-Dieter: Der Garten als Mikrokosmos, Hermann Bauer, Freiburg im Breisgau 1982.

Thakkur, Ch. G.: Ayurveda, Hermann Bauer, Freiburg im Breisgau 1977.

Thomas, P.: Hindu Religion, Customs and Manners, Taraporevala sons & Co, Bombay 1971.

Todamanda: Materia Medica of Ayurveda, based on Ayurveda Saukhyam of Todarananda, Naurang Rai, New Delhi 1980.

Tompkins, P./Bird, Ch.: Das geheime Leben der Pflanzen, Scherz, Bern—München 1973.

Udupa, K.N./Tripathi, S. N.: Natürliche Heilkräfte, F. P. Schwitter Holding AG, Zürich 1980.

Vagabhata: Astangha Hrdaya Samhita, E. J. Brill, Leiden 1941.

Vithaloas, Yogi: Das Yoga Kochbuch, Heyne, München 1977.

Weck, Wolfgang: Heilkunde und Volkstum auf Bali, P. T. BAP. Pali, P. T. Intermasa, Jakarta, 1976.

Willfort, Richard: Gesundheit durch Heilkräuter, Rudolf Trauner, Linz 1979.

Wong, Ming: Handbuch der chinesischen Pflanzenheilkunde, Hermann Bauer, Freiburg im Breisgau 1978.

GLOSSARY OF SANSKRIT WORDS

Adraka — fresh ginger, *Zingiber officinalis*

Agada Tantra — treatise on poisoings

agneya — fiery

Agneya — the hot half of the year

Agni — fire; biological combustion

Agni mantha — *Prema integrifolia*

Agnivesa Samhita — medical text

Aguru — *Aquilaria agallocha*

Ahamkara — ego; personality

Ahara rasa — chyle; food juice

Akasha — ether; space

Akasiya — relating to ether or space

Akriti — general impression, face

Alocaka Pitta — a variety of *Pitta Dosha*

ama — unripe; undigested

Amajanya — endogenous diseases

Amalaki — *Emblica officinalis*

Amara — *Mangifera indica*; mango

Amavata — form of disease in which *Agni* misfunctions

amla — sour

Amlika — *Tamarindus indica*

Analanama — *Plumbago ceylanico*

Anna — therapy form

Anna Vaha Srotas — channels

Anupana — type of landscape

Anurasa — fugitive flavor

Anuvasana — oily enemata

Ap — water

Apana Vata — a variety of *Vata Dosha*

apya — watery

Arjuna — *Terminalia arjuna*

Arka — *Calotropis gigantea*

Arista — fermented vegetable extract

Asana — a posture in Hatha Yoga

Astanga Sangraha — a medical text

Astanga Hridaya — a medical text

Asthi — constituents of bone tissue

Asvattha — *Ficus religiosa*

Atharva Veda — one of the four most ancient philosphical and religious writings of India

Ativisa — *Aconitum heterophyllum*

Atman — *Purusha* (q.v.)

Ausadha — medicines

Avalambaka Kapha — a variety of *Kapha Dosha*

Babula — *Acacia catechu*

Bakuchi — *Psoralea corylifolia*

Bala — *Sida cordifolia*

Bala Tantra — pediatrics and gynecology

Bhallataka — *Semencarpus anacardium*

Bhasmaka — form of disease in

which *Agni* is defective

Bhava Prakasa — medical text

Bheda — the sixth of the 'six stages of disease

Bhrajaka Pitta — a variety of *Pitta Dosha*

Bhutagni — five forms of the biological fire *Agni*

Bhuta Vidya — the treatment of mental troubles by animistic spirits, mantras, and tantras

Bibhitaki — *Terminalia belerica*

Bida Lavana — a kind of rock salt

Bilva — *Aegle marmalos*

Bodhaka Kapha — a variety of *Kapha Dosha*

Brahma — a Hindu divinity

Brahmins — members of the priestly caste

Brahmi — 1. *Bacopa monieri*; 2. *Centella asiatica*

Brihati — *Solanum indicum*

Brimhana — a form of therapy

Buddhi — intellect; understanding

Cangeri — *Oxalis acetosella*

Charaka Samhita — a medical work

Cavya — *Piper cubeba*

Chitraka — *Plumbago ceylanica*

Dadima — *Punica granatum*; pomegranate

Darbha — *Imperata cylindrica*

Dasa Mula — the 'ten roots'

Dharana — concentration of the mind in Yoga

Dhataki — *Woodfordia fructicosa*

Dhatu — the 'tissues' supporting the body

Dhatu Agni — seven forms of *Agni*

Dhyana — meditation [rather: sustained concentration]

Dosha — labile balance of a bioenergetic principle; one of

the three forces governing all biological processes

Draksa — *Vitis vinifera*; the grape-vine

drava — liquid

Dravya — substance

Dravyaguna — pharmacology and pharmacognoscy

Drika — the eyes

Gamhara — *Gmelina arborea*

Grisma — mid-May to mid-July

Guggulu — *Commiphora mukul*

Guna — 1. Elementary property of primordial matter; 2. Quality or property in general

guru — heavy

Haridra — *Curcuma longa*

Haritaki — *Terminalia chebula*

Hemanta — mid-November to mid-January

Hingu — *Ferula narthex*

Iksu — *Saccharum officinarum*; cane sugar

Jala — water

Jangala — a type of landscape

Jatamansi — *Nardochstachys jatamansi*

Jathahara Agni — a form of *Agni*

Jati — *Jasminum grandiflorum*

Jatiphala — *Myristica fragrans*; nutmeg; mace

Jihva — *tongue*

Jiva — *Atman*; *Purusha*

Kantakari — *Solanum xanthocarpium*

Kapha Dosha — bioenergetic principle

Karma — action; movement

Kasa — *Saccharum spontaneum*

kasaya — astringent
Kasmiri — *Sausurea lappa*
kathina — hard
katu — pungent
Katuka — *Picrorhiza kurroa*
Kaya chikitsa — internal medicine
Kebuka — *Costus speciosus*
Khajura — *Phoenix sylvestris*; date palm
khara — rough
Khorpara — copra
Kledaka Kapha — a variety of *Kapha Dosha*
Kolpra vriksa — *Cocus nucifera*; coconut tree
Krishna — a Hindu divinity
Kshatriyas — members of the warrior caste
Kumari — *Aloe barbadensis*
Kupilu — *Strychnos nux vomica*
Kusa — *Demostachy bipinata*
Kustha — *Saussurea lappa*
Kutaja — *Holarrhena antidysenterica*
Kutaki — *Picrorhiza kurroa*

laghu — light
Langhana — a form of therapy
Lavana — salt
lavana — salty

Madhava Nidana — a medical text
Madhu — honey
madhura — sweet
Mahabharata — Indian national epic
Mahabhuta — primordial element; one of the building blocks of being
Majja — component of bone marrow
Majja Vaha Srotas — ducts
Malas — waste materials of the body

Malam — feces
Mamsa — component of muscle
Mamsa Vaha Srotas — ducts
Manas — mind; spirit
manda — milk; slow; inert
Mandagni — a form of *Agni*
Mandukarpani — *Centalla asiatica*
Marica — *Piper nigrum*; black pepper
Meda — component of fat
Meda Vaha Srotas — ducts
Medhya Rasayan — mind-expanding drugs
mridu — soft
Mutra — urine
Mutra Vaha Srota — duct

Nadi — pulse
Nimba — *Azadirachta indica*
Niruhana — dry, cleansing enemata
Niyama — Yoga doctrine of body care
Nyaya Vaisheshika — a system of psychological and logical categories

Ojas Dhatu — the total ambience of an individual formed from the sum of the seven *Dhatus*

Pachaka Pitta — a variety of *Pitta Dosha*
Palandu — *Allium cepa*; onion
Pancha Karma — five cleansing therapies
Pancha Mahabhutas — the five primoridal elements
Pancha Nimba — the five parts of the *Nimba* tree
Pancha Trina Mula — the roots of the 'five grasses'
Pariahs — pariahs or outcasts
Paribhadraka — *Erythrina indica*
prathiva — earthy
Patala — *Stereospermum sauveolens*

picchila — slimy

Pippali — *Piper longum*

Pitta Dosha — the bioenergetic principle

Prabhava — pharmacological drug action

Prakopa — excitement or stimulation

Prakriti — nature matter

Prana Vata — a variety of *Vata Dosha*

Prana Vaha Srotas — ducts

Pranayama — the regulation of breath as taught in Yoga

Prasara — spreading

Pratyahara — Yoga teaching concerning the 'stilling' of the senses and thoughts

Prthivi — earth

Purisha — feces

Purisha Vaha Srota — a duct

Purusha — 1. the human self; 2. the universal spirit principle

Rajas — the energy principle; a property of primordial matter

Rajika — *Brassica nigra*; mustard

Rajsik — one of the three categories of nourishment in Buddhist *Sattwik* teaching

Raksha — a demon

Rakta Dhatu — component of the blood

Raktu Vaha Srotas — ducts

Ranjaka Pitta — a variety of *Pitta Dosha*

Rasa — taste

Rasa Dhatu — component of blood plasma

Rasa Vaha Srotas — ducts

Rasayan — rejuvenating substances

Rasayan Tantra — geriatrics

Rasona — *Allium sativum*; garlic

Rigveda — the oldest Indian philosophical and religious work

Romaka Lavana — a type of salt

ruksa — dry

Ruksana — a form of therapy

Sadhaka Pitta — a variety of *Pitta Dosha*

Saindhava Lavana — rock salt

Salakya Tantra — treatment of the ears, nose, throat, eyes, jaws, and teeth

Salaparni — *Desmodium gangeticum*

Sali — *Oryza sativa*; rice

Sallaki — *Boswellia serrata*

Salya Tantra — surgery

Samadhi — raptness [in the object of contemplation]

Samagni — a form of *Agni*

Samana Vata — a variety of *Vata Dosha*

Samanya — sameness; genus

Samavaya — inseparable inherence

Samaveda — one of the oldest Indian philosophical and religious writings

Sambhava Lavana — saline efflorescence on oil

Samkhya — a school of philosophy

samsamana — symptomatic; calming; palliative

Samsodhana — causal; cleansing; radical

Samtapraa — group of disorders in which *Agni* is misfunctioning

Samudra — sea salt

Sancaya — congestion; accumulation

sandra — solid; dense

Saptaparna — *Alstonia scholaris*

sara — mobile

Sarpagandha — *Rauwolfia serpentina*

Sata Kriyakala — the six stages of disease

Satavari — *Asparagus racemosus*

Sattwa — essence; the spiritual principle of prime matter

Sattvik — Buddhist dietary doctrine

Saumya — the cold time of year; the moon

Sauvarcala Lavana — a type of rock salt

Shabda — voice

Shalmali — *Bombax malabaricum*

Shankhapuspi — *Convulvulus pluricaulis*

Sharad — the season from mid-September to mid-November

Shisira — the season from mid-January to mid-March

Shirisa — *Albizzia lebbek*

Shiva — a Hindu divinity

Shudras — members of the servant caste

Sirovirechana — cleansing therapy for the head

sita — cool; cold

slaksna — smooth

Slesaka Kapha — a form of *Kapha Dosha*

Slesma — *Kapha*; cementing

Snehana — a form of therapy

snigdha — oily

Sparsa — skin

Srota — canal; body duct

Stambhana — a form of therapy

Stana Samsraya — localization

sthira — compact; static

sthula — gross

Sugandha Bala — *Valeriana wallichi*

Sukra Dhatu — components of the male semen or female ova

Sukra Dhatu Srotas — ducts

suksma — minute; fine

Sunthi — dried ginger; *Zingiber officinalis*

Susruta Samhita — a medical work

Sweda — sweat; perspiration

Sweda Vaha Srotas — ducts

Swedana — a therapy form

Syonaka — *Droxylum indicum*

Tagara — *Valeriana wallichi*

taijasa — fiery

Taila — sesame oil

Tamaka's Swasa — bronchial asthma

Tamas — mass; the principle of materiality; a property of prime matter

Tambula — *Piper betle*; betel nut

Tamsik — one of the three categories of nourishment in *Sattwik* doctrine

Tarpaka Kapha — a variety of *Kapha Dosha*

Tejas — fire

tiksna — keen, pungent

Tiksnagni — one of the four constituent forms of *Agni*

tikta — bitter

Tri Doshas — the three bioenergetic principles

Trikatu — the 'three pungents'

Tri Phala — the 'three fruits'

Tulsi — *Ocimum sanctum*

Tuvaraka — *Hydnocarpus wightiana*

Udana Vata — a form of *Vata Dosha*

Udaka Vaha Srotas — ducts

Udumbara — *Ficus racemosa*

Upanishads — later additions to the Vedas

Upasaya — therapy

Usira — *Vetivera zizanoides*

usna — hot

Vacha — *Acorus calamus*; sweet calamus

Vaisyas — members of the merchant caste

Vajikarana Tantra — sexual lore

Vamana — emetics

Varsa — season from mid-July to mid-September

Vasa — *Adhatoda vasica*

Vasanta — season from mid-March to mid-May

Vata Dosha — bioenergetic principle

Vata — *Ficus bengaliensis*; banyan tree

Vatarakta — disorder in which *Agni* misfunctions

Vatsanabha — *Aconitum ferox*

vayayva — windy

Vayu — air

Vidanga — *Embelia ribes*

Vidari — *Ipomea paniculata*

Vihara — a form of therapy

Vipaka — taste of digested, transformed nourishment

Virecana — purging

Virya — healing potency

visada — clear; transparent

Visamagni — a form of *Agni*

Visesa — diversity

Vishnu — a Hindu divinity

vyakti — excited; the stage of manifestation

Vyana Vata — a form of *Vata Dosha*

Yajurveda — one of the four oldest philosophical and religious writings of India

Yama — Yoga teaching on social behavior

Yastimadhu — *Glycyrrhiza glabra*; liquorice

Yogaratnakara — the eightfold method of investigation

INDEXES

Index of English Plant Names

Medical Index